T0215843

FAST FACTS for
THE ADULT-GERONTOLOGY ACUTE CARE NURSE PRACTITIONER

Dawn Carpenter, DNP, ACNP-BC, CCRN, is a practicing acute care nurse practitioner with the trauma and surgical service line at Guthrie Healthcare System in Pennsylvania. In addition, she is an associate professor at her alma mater, the University of Massachusetts Medical School, Graduate School of Nursing. She currently mentors DNP students, teaches an elective course on living with chronic and terminal illness, and is the former coordinator of the adult-gerontology acute care nurse practitioner program. Dr. Carpenter possesses a passion for educating acute and critical care nurses and nurse practitioners and has 30 years of experience as a critical care nurse, nurse practitioner, and faculty member.

Dr. Carpenter mentored many new NPs, postgraduate residents, and new hires throughout her career and consistently noted how each of them would keep a notebook with tidbits of information for handy recall. Hence the concept to publish this book was born.

Dr. Carpenter is actively engaged at the national level with the American Association of Critical Care Nurses, where she routinely volunteers her time and expertise. She has served as a volunteer item writer for the ACNPC-AG exam and as a member of the exam development committee for the ACNPC-AG and CCRN exams. She is the current cochair of the Advanced Practice Institute (API) planning committee.

FAST FACTS for
THE ADULT-GERONTOLOGY ACUTE CARE NURSE PRACTITIONER

Dawn Carpenter, DNP, ACNP-BC, CCRN

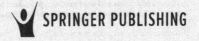 SPRINGER PUBLISHING

Springer Publishing Company, LLC
11 West 42nd Street, New York, NY 10036
www.springerpub.com
connect.springerpub.com

Acquisitions Editor: Rachel X. Landes
Compositor: Transforma

ISBN: 978-0-8261-5204-6
ebook ISBN: 978-0-8261-5224-4
DOI: 10.1891/9780826152244

21 22 23 24/ 5 4 3 2 1

The author and the publisher of this Work have made every effort to use sources believed to be reliable
to provide information that is accurate and compatible with the standards generally accepted at the
time of publication. Because medical science is continually advancing, our knowledge base continues
to expand. Therefore, as new information becomes available, changes in procedures become necessary.
We recommend that the reader always consult current research and specific institutional policies before
performing any clinical procedure or delivering any medication. The author and publisher shall not
be liable for any special, consequential, or exemplary damages resulting, in whole or in part, from the
readers' use of, or reliance on, the information contained in this book. The publisher has no responsibility for the persistence or accuracy of URLs for external or third-party internet websites referred to in
this publication and does not guarantee that any content on such websites is, or will remain, accurate
or appropriate.

Library of Congress Cataloging-in-Publication Data
LCCN: 2021058304

Publisher's Note: **New and used products purchased from third-party sellers are not guaranteed for
quality, authenticity, or access to any included digital components.**

Printed in the United States of America.

This book is dedicated to all current AG-ACNP students, newly minted AG-ACNPs, as well as seasoned AG-ACNPs. I am inspired by your commitment and dedication to the profession. You have been the nidus to publish this book. It is a compilation of what many of you have collected in your own handwritten notebooks. These books have given me insights into what information is needed at your fingertips, as you onboard to new clinical rotations and embark upon your careers. I am eager to hear what else should be included for the next edition.

Contents

Part III SPECIAL POPULATIONS

Part IV SPECIAL CONSIDERATIONS FOR ADVANCED PRACTICE ACUTE CARE NURSING

Content Reviewers

Jennifer Adamski, DNP, APRN, ACNP-BC, CCRN, FCCM, Assistant Professor, AG-ACNP Program Director, Critical Care Nurse Practitioner, Emory University, Atlanta, Georgia; ACNP Critical Care Nurse Practitioner, Critical Care Flight Team, Cleveland Clinic, Cleveland, Ohio

Kathleen Ballman, DNP, ACNP-BC, CEN, Associate Professor of Clinical Nursing, Coordinator of Adult-Gerontology Acute Care Nurse Practitioner Program, University of Cincinnati, College of Nursing, Cincinnati, Ohio

Leanne H. Fowler, DNP, MBA, AGACNP-BC, CNE, Assistant Professor of Clinical Nursing, Director of Nurse Practitioner Programs, Coordinator of Adult Gerontology Acute Care NP Concentration, LSU Health New Orleans School of Nursing, New Orleans, Louisiana

Stefanie La Manna, PhD, MPH, APRN, FNP-C, AGACNP-BC, Associate Professor, Department Chair of Graduate Programs, Ron and Kathy Assaf College of Nursing, Nova Southeastern University, Palm Beach Gardens, Florida

Alexander Menard, DNP, AGACNP-BC, Assistant Professor, Coordinator AG-ACNP track, Graduate School of Nursing, University of Massachusetts Medical School, Worcester, Massachusetts

Kelsey O'Brien, M.Div., Chaplain to Palliative Care and Special Pathogens ICU, Penn State Hershey Medical Center, Hershey, Pennsylvania

Mimi Pomerleau, DNP, MPH, RNC-OB, RNC-MNN, C-ONQS, CNE, Professional Development Manager, Brigham and Women's Hospital, Boston, Massachusetts

Erica Smeltz, MS, CRNP, NPC, Palliative Care Nurse Practitioner, Penn State Hershey Medical Center, Hershey, Pennsylvania

Mike Spiros, MALD, MS, APRN, AGACNP-BC, Nurse Manager, Medical Intensive Care Unit, Mayo Clinic, Jacksonville, Florida

Kimberly Taylor, MS, AG-ACNP, Cardiology Nurse Practitioner, UMass Memorial Medical Center, Instructor, University of Massachusetts Medical School, Graduate School of Nursing, Worcester, Massachusetts

Preface

Welcome to the first edition of *Fast Facts for the Adult-Gerontology Acute Care Nurse Practitioner* book. This book was created specifically for AG-ACNP students and new hires as well as for NPs who are changing positions or moving to a new organization. This book presents critical information at the NP's fingertips for quick reference in clinical settings.

This book is designed to be kept in the pocket of a lab coat or handy on a computer on wheels. It is designed to be used during clinical rotations and in everyday practice. AG-ACNPs can use this book as review material for exams, a reference in clinical or simulation settings, writing case studies, and applying to patient care while in practice.

This book is unique in that it provides many tables and charts to provide large amounts of data in a condensed format. Given the expansive knowledge that AG-ACNPs must know, it was impossible to include everything and yet be small enough for the pocket, thus selective components were chosen for inclusion.

I am eager to receive feedback on this book so that we can create a superior second edition. Any suggestions, additions, or critiques can be sent to Dawn Carpenter at Dawn.Carpenter@umassmed.edu.

Dawn Carpenter

Acknowledgments

I want to extend my sincerest gratitude to my colleagues Jennifer Gramley and Jackie Thoryk, who have selflessly shared the content in their homemade books, which motivated me.

Thank you to Elizabeth Nieginski and Rachel Landes at Springer Publishing Company for providing me the opportunity to publish this book. You have been so very graciously patient with me during the COVID-19 pandemic. You are amazing partners, and I am humbled by your confidence in me to accomplish this goal.

Most importantly, I am eternally grateful to my loving husband, Andy, who has unwaveringly and selflessly supported my career. You have provided infinite love, patience, and sustenance to help make this book a reality—I love you!

Introduction

Congratulations! Whether you are an AG-ACNP student who is embarking into clinical, newly graduated beginning your first position, or an experienced AG-ACNP starting employment caring for a new population, this book will be a handy pocket resource for you. This book is designed to be a quick reference with helpful information in an easy-to-access format. It has quick tips on medication dosing, ordering diagnostic tests, documentation, and billing. Most importantly, many fine nuances and quick tips for each body system are included. While your AG-ACNP program provided a solid foundation, many important details cannot be memorized and take time and repetition to engrain into daily practice.

This book does not replace textbooks, clinical practice guidelines, or comprehensive reading and studying. To apply the concepts in this book, one requires a broader and deeper understanding of the pathophysiology, diagnoses, and treatments of diverse acute, acute on chronic, and critical care conditions.

About this book:
This book is intended for

- AG-ACNP students who are in clinical rotations,
- newly graduated AG-ACNPs who are starting their first AG-ACNP position, and
- experienced AG-ACNPs who are starting a new position with a different population.

Faculty can utilize this book

- as an adjunct to case-based discussions in the classroom,
- as a resource for students in high-fidelity simulations,

- as a pocket resource to support students in clinical rotations, and
- to equip new graduates to function more efficiently in practice

Postgraduate residencies and fellowships can utilize this book

- to augment education of AG-ACNPs and
- to empower independent, safe decision-making.

I

Adult-Gerontology Acute Care Nurse Practitioner

1

Organizing the Shift

Getting organized and staying organized throughout the shift are critical to providing care. And caring for acutely and critically ill patients requires flexibility to meet the patient and organizational needs. Some days start by seeing the most critical patients first to provide stabilization, while other shifts require discharging or transferring stable patients to make room for higher acuity patients. Thus, no two days are exactly the same. The key is having situational awareness and adjusting the routine accordingly. Communication with the charge nurse is critical to understanding the unit and institutional needs.

In this chapter, you will learn

- how to organize yourself to enhance efficiency,
- a system of how to give and receive the handoff,
- how to triage patients,
- a systematic method to preround on your patients, and
- techniques to ensure follow-up on actionable items.

ORGANIZE YOURSELF FIRST

A key step is to develop an organizational process that works for you. Observe the workflow of your preceptors, and try out a few different styles to see what is most comfortable for you. A typical shift for any provider is to receive a patient list or handoff tool with clinical data. These vary in form and amount of data, some are simply a list of names and diagnoses, where others contain problem lists, laboratory data, medication lists, and

Table 1.1

Example Patient List						
Room #	Name, MRN	Code status	Reason for admission and significant PMH	24-hour events	Active problems and treatments	To Do

MRN, medical record number; PMH, past medical history.

code status. Working with an existing list or creating your own hand-off tool is acceptable. Knowing what important data is needed to provide care for the patient is essential and may be unique to your practice. Table 1.1 is an example of a typical list and how to organize data in a meaningful way to focus on the patient's top priorities.

Once you have this handoff data, which is a cursory overview, additional details are needed to develop a comprehensive plan. For some, the next step is to perform chart reviews, then go examine patients, while others prefer the visual aspect of seeing the patient and talking with nursing staff and then review the chart. The latter process is helpful in that the nurse practitioner (NP) can address any pressing issues immediately. Communicating early in the shift with the nurse is also an opportunity to gather critical information about social aspects that are not readily found in the chart. There is no right or wrong system, but having one process and adhering to it is central to quality care.

As you examine the patient, review medications, and formally round on the patient, keep adding to the "To Do" column of the handoff tool. Refer to this list on an hourly basis throughout the day. As items are completed or diagnostic test results are reviewed, check these off the list and write down the results. Keeping track of the plan for the patient in this manner is helpful in three important ways:

1. Helps you to ensure actionable items get completed.
2. Enhances efficiency and ensures thorough and complete documentation.
3. Aids in providing a comprehensive handoff to the next team or shift.

Fast Facts

Never delay any task. Get the work done as soon as possible so you are prepared for the next thing that comes up, be it an admission, a code, or an impromptu discharge. This state of readiness will pay off at the end of the day, when you get out on time, thus enhancing your quality of life.

HANDOFF

Giving and receiving a handoff can be challenging to master as a new NP. When receiving handoff, a large quantity of data is conveyed in a short amount of time. Knowing which details will need to be recalled at a later point can be difficult, in addition to learning how to sift through this voluminous auditory data and to know what to write down. Thus, many NPs initially write down everything they hear in handoff. Many NPs find that writing things down helps them remember better. Helpful tips include circling or highlighting key data on the list and learning how to abbreviate your notes, both of which save time writing. Common things easy to abbreviate:

- ventilator modes and settings
- sedatives
- positive cultures
- antibiotics

Giving a handoff report can be a daunting task. A lot of information needs to be condensed into a few sentences to accurately and concisely convey the status of the patient for continuity of care. This requires practice to give sufficient information efficiently, not too much and yet, not too little that significant problems get overlooked (see Table 1.2). The key is to articulate in medical diagnoses, rather than symptoms.

Critical content to communicate to the receiver during a handoff should include:

- sender contact information
- illness assessment, including severity

Table 1.2

Comparison of Two Brief Handoff Reports

Novice Handoff:	Expert:
75-year-old man with a history of hypertension, coronary artery disease, hyperlipidemia, and MI 4 months ago s/p stent. He presented with 2-day history of SOB, and today developed fever and chills and a cough. At about noon he developed worsening shortness of breath and coughed up yellow phlegm. He has one sick contact, his granddaughter, whom was home sick from daycare. CXR showed right lower lobe infiltrate. White count was 14. He became hypoxic to 80% on a non-rebreather mask and then was intubated. He became hypotensive to 90s with intubation medications but has since recovered and is back to his normal of 130/70. His BUN and Creatinine are elevated and he received 2 L IVF in the emergency department. Blood cultures and sputum cultures were sent.	Mr. Smith is 75 years old, Full Code, was admitted today with acute hypoxic respiratory failure d/t CAP. Course c/b AKI likely d/t dehydration with ongoing hydration. PMH significant for: HTN, and an MI 4 months ago s/p stent. F/U sputum gram stain; Chem 7 pending at 2,200, taper fluids tonight. Vent is at 60% and 8 Peep – wean to 40% then Peep to five for sat >92%. Restart ACEi when creatinine normalizes.

(continued)

Table 1.2

Comparison of Two Brief Handoff Reports (*continued*)

Novice Handoff:	Expert:
Assessment: This is a great start to an HPI, but too long for a handoff. However, it forces the reader to synthesize the same data to come to the same diagnosis, so it's easier to just state the diagnosis.	Assessment: Summarizes with good use of medical terminology to concisely articulate the patient's current status. Outlines plan for the night shift to continue patient's recovery. However, it is still missing a few key factors. See below:

ACEi, angiotension-converting-enzyme inhibitor; AKI, acute kidney injury; CAP, community acquired pneumonia; CXR, chest x-ray; HPI, history of present illness; HTN, hypertension; MI, myocardial infarction; PMH, past medical history; SOB, shortness of breath.

- Patient summary, including events leading up to illness or admission, hospital course, ongoing assessment, and plan of care
- To-do action list
- Contingency plans
- Allergy list
- Code status
- Medication list
- Dated laboratory tests
- Dated vital signs

Multiple mnemonics for handoff exist.
SBAR

- Situation
- Background
- Assessment
- Recommendation

I-PASS

- Illness severity
- Patient summary
- Action list
- Situation awareness and contingency plans
- Synthesis by receiver

I PUT PATIENTS FIRST

- Identify yourself and role and obtain nurse's name
- Patient's past medical history (medical, surgical, social)
- Underlying diagnosis and procedure
- Technique (general anesthesia, neuraxial, regional)
- Peripheral IVs, arterial lines, central lines, drains
- Allergies
- Therapeutic interventions (pain medications, antibiotics)

- Intubation (very difficult, moderately difficult, easy)
- Extubation likelihood (already extubated, very likely, unlikely, definitely no extubation planned)
- Need for drips (epinephrine, vasopressin, norepinephrine, insulin, propofol, etc.)
- Treatment plan for postoperative care (blood pressure goals, ventilator settings)
- Signs (vital signs during case and most recent)
- Fluids (ins and outs, blood product(s) administered)
- Intraoperative events (if any)
- Recent labs (hemoglobin, glucose, etc.)
- Suggestions for immediate postop care (special positioning, pain control, need for pumps, etc.)
- Timing/expected time of arrival to ICU

TRIAGE

Part of the NP role is to triage the patient's level of acuity and get the patient to the level of care that matches their current needs (see Table 1.3). Identifying which patients meet ICU, step-down, or floor level of care is done on an ongoing basis. In addition, NPs routinely make decisions regarding who can be discharged to long-term acute care hospitals (LTACH), acute rehabilitation, skilled nursing facilities, and home with services. In community hospitals, the NP also makes decisions to transfer patients to tertiary and/or quaternary care centers. The biggest factors in making these decisions are patient acuity combined with the nursing and institutional/facility capabilities.

Before rushing to judgment and making decisions regarding patients, take time to become familiar with the admission, discharge, and transfer (ADT) criteria within the institution, and then seek to gain an understanding of the capabilities of the local facilities where patients are discharged to within the community. Practice patterns vary between regions of the country. A patient who may be too sick to stay in a community hospital's ICU may only meet the step-down level of care in a tertiary hospital. Conversely, patients who may be too sick to send to a floor may not be sick enough to send to an LTACH.

ROUNDS

Morning

Upon getting the report, the NP will preround on their patients, which includes

- reviewing objective data,
- performing a physical exam and interview the patient,
- talking with the nurse, and
- developing a preliminary plan.

Table 1.3

Levels of Care

Level of care	Type of care	Nurse-to-patient ratio	Care provided
Intensive care unit	Critically ill patients who need hourly and/or invasive and continuous monitoring	1:1 or 1:2	Invasive interventions, including invasive mechanical ventilation, vasopressor titration, CRRT, ICP monitoring and drainage, ECMO, IABP, VAD
Intermediate care unit	Unstable patients who need nursing interventions, lab workup and/or monitoring every 2–4 hours.	≤1:3	Interventions such as noninvasive ventilation, IV infusions, titrations of vasodilators or antiarrhythmics
Telemetry (if hospitals do not have this level of care, admit to next higher level)	Stable patients who require monitoring of electrocardiographic for nonmalignant arrhythmias; VS not more frequent than every 2–4 hours	≤1:4	IV infusions and titrations of medications such as vasodilators or antiarrhythmics
General care floor	Stable patients who need monitoring and testing not more frequently than every 2–4 hours	≤1:5	IV antibiotics, IV chemotherapy, laboratory, and/or radiographic studies

CRRT, continuous renal replacement therapy; ECMO, extracorporeal membrane oxygenation; IABP, intra-aortic balloon pump; ICP, intracranial pressure; VAD, ventricular assist device; VS, vital signs.

On formal rounds, the plan of the day is refined with input from other members of the team. The NP can be instrumental in actively engaging nursing, respiratory therapists, pharmacist, nutritionist, case management, social work, and others, such as palliative care, and physical or occupational/speech therapy as patient status dictates.

Afternoon

After formal rounds, the NP should round at least once in the afternoon to

- reassess patients again,
- review results from testing that was completed,
- assess response to interventions and assess for additional tweaks to the plan of care,
- determine if additional interventions or changes to management plans are needed, and
- update family on the plan if they were not included in formal morning rounds.

Fast Facts

Rerounding periodically throughout the day, to reexamine the patient and speak with the nurse throughout the shift is critical to staying on top of ever-changing patient status. It allows real-time response to changes in condition.

Evening

Many NPs work 12-hour shifts, thus when the oncoming night team receives the handoff, they too should make rounds. Again, review data; review vital signs; assess IV fluids and infusions, ventilator settings, intake/output, lab data; and seek to see if any additional weaning can occur or if a diet or activity can be advanced, or conversely, if the patient's condition is worsening, requiring additional interventions and escalation of care. Patients continually change, and it's up to the NP to actively engage to promote health.

Fast Facts

Continually seek to find small ways to move the patient closer to the door. In other words, what can be done to ready the patient for discharge. Seek to minimize interventions by discontinuing the urinary catheter, decrease or saline-lock IV fluids, progress mobility status, advance diet, order physical therapy, and so forth.

Middle of the Night

Sleep is critical to healing and the prevention of delirium; thus, assessment of sleep and promotion of sleep hygiene are crucial elements of the NP role.

- Observe the patient from the doorway.
- Seek to engage nursing staff to dim lights.

- Advocate for a quiet environment.
- Offer the patient eye masks and ear plugs.
- Turn off the TVs and music.
- Avoid medications that are known to be delirogenic (e.g., benzodiazepines, diphenhydramine, zolpidem).
- Perform chart reviews to monitor patient.

The night shift is a great time for providers to update the ICU and/or hospital course and discharge summary to start the discharge planning documentation. If the hospital course summary is kept up to date, the oncoming or receiving team will have succinct information to immediately assume care of the patient.

FOLLOW-UP AND REASSESSMENT

The NP is responsible to follow up on results of diagnostic testing; input and recommendations from consultants; and assessment of the plans and interventions from the plan of the day.

Calling Consults

Consultants offer feedback specifically on the clinical question that is posed to them. Be sure to have a clear clinical question or problem that they are to answer when you call a consult. Use of the situation, background, assessment, and recommendation (SBAR) communication process is useful to concisely describe the patient circumstances and request input from a consultant provider. Critically appraise the recommendations:

- Do the recommendations make sense?
- Do these recommendations align with the overall plan laid out by the primary team?
- If there are any questions, discrepancies or conflicts should be discussed with the primary team.

Triage Diagnostic Testing and Therapeutic Interventions

The NP is responsible to follow up on diagnostic testing results and/or therapeutic interventions. Commonly, NPs need to negotiate with other departments to prioritize tests that are critical to making a diagnosis or to decide on a treatment plan. Triaging the urgency of diagnostic testing and balancing the risks associated with that testing and the travel for testing can be challenging. Knowing when to push to get things done versus when to say something can be delayed can be challenging. Seek input from the other team members, and make collective decisions. If a critically ill patient who is at high risk to travel, needs to travel, the NP should travel with the nurse and patient.

Chart Reviews

Acutely and critically ill patient conditions are ever evolving, some in a positive direction, some in a negative direction. Hourly chart rounding is essential to watch for trends in improvement or deterioration. Don't wait for the nurse to call; be proactive. Staying abreast of this evolving care is critical to early identification of actual or impending problems and preventing or mitigating larger problems.

Fast Facts

Be proactive. Don't wait for the nurse to call you about a change in patient condition.

In summary, organize yourself first. Have a system to track data and tasks to improve efficiency. Continuous evaluation and modification of the plan of care during a shift is imperative.

References

Chapman, Y. L. (2016). Nurse satisfaction with information technology enhanced bedside handoff. *MedSurg Nursing*, *25*(5), 313–318.

Haig, K. M., Sutton, S., & Whittington, J. (2006). SBAR: A shared mental model for improving communication between clinicians. *The Joint Commission Journal on Quality and Patient Safety*, *32*(3), 167–175.

Moon, T. S., Gonzales, M. X., & Woods, A. P. (2015). A mnemonic to facilitate the handover from the operating room to intensive care unit: "I PUT PATIENTS FIRST." *Journal of Anesthesia and Clinical Research*, *6*(7), 545.

Nates, J. L., Nunnally, M., Kleinpell, R., Blosser, S., Goldner, J., Birriel, B., Fowler, C. S., Byrum, D., Miles, W. S., Bailey, H., & Sprung, C. L. (2016). ICU admission, discharge, and triage guidelines: A framework to enhance clinical operations, development of institutional policies, and further research. *Critical Care Medicine*, *44*(8), 1553–1602. https://doi.org/10.1097/ccm.0000000000001856

Smith, S. T., Enderby, S. F., Bessler, R. A. (2017). Teamwork in leadership and practice-based management. In S. C. Editor McKean, J. J. Ross, D. D. Dressler, D. B. Scheurer (Eds.), *Principles and practice of hospital medicine* (2 ed., pp. 157–170). McGraw Hill Education.

Starmer, A. J., Spector, N. D., Srivastava, R., Allen, A. D., Landrigan, C. P., Sectish, T. C., & I-PASS Study Group. (2012). I-PASS, a mnemonic to standardize verbal handoffs. *Pediatrics*, *129*(2), 201–204.

The Joint Commission. (2017, September 12, 2017). *Sentinel Event Alert: Inadequate hand-off communication*. Joint Commission. www.e-handoff.com/wp-content/uploads/2017/09/Joint-Commission-Handoff-Communication-Alert.pdf

2

Who and When to Call for Help

Caring for acutely and critically ill patients is truly a team sport. Everyone brings expertise to the bedside. Recognizing the strengths and limitations of other team members and utilizing their expertise are what promote excellent patient outcomes. We simultaneously need to recognize our own limitations and know when to ask for help. We cannot be afraid or too proud to ask for help.

In this chapter, you will learn

- to take a personal inventory of your strengths and limitations,
- to identify your human and institutional resources and how to contact them,
- what types of situations require escalation up the chain of command, and
- which situations require the attending physician to be notified.

KNOW YOURSELF

Personal Inventory

The first and most important task is to take a personal inventory of your individual strengths, including nursing experience, AG-ACNP experience, and technical skills.

- Review clinical areas in which you are strong, and acknowledge your limitations.
- On your time off, read texts and review articles first to gain an overview, then read the clinical practice guidelines, and, finally, peruse current research articles.

- Don't be shy. Ask colleagues to review pathophysiology, diagnostics, and management of the conditions when it applies to patients under your care.

Ask about resources to hone your technical and procedural skills. Do you have access to a simulation center or other departments that do a lot of procedures to refine these skills? Advocate for yourself when opportunities arise so that you can build your skill mix.

Self-Awareness and Self-Reflection

Critical to success as an AG-ACNP is self-awareness and self-reflection. Be aware of interpersonal interactions, including communications among staff and team members. Assess the verbal message—what are you saying? Reflect upon how it is being perceived, and did the receiver hear the message clearly? Closed-loop communication is paramount to patient safety. Nonverbal language, including posture, voice tone, hesitancy or curtness, facial expressions, and so forth, conveys a host of emotions, such as anxiety, insecurity, and frustration, among others. These interpersonal interactions can either build the team's respect and trust of you or devalue your contributions. AG-ACNPs need to be able to self-reflect on interactions with staff and team members to evaluate the impact on the team. Additionally, the NP must be open to feedback. If feedback is not provided, the NP should ask for feedback to augment clinical and team performance.

Fast Facts

You may need to specifically ask teammates for feedback to enhance and augment your clinical knowledge and performance. Sample questions: How am I doing? On what areas do I need to focus? What would you have me do differently in managing that patient or situation? Any suggestions to improve?

Situational Awareness

Hospitalized patients can shift from acutely to critically ill in minutes, and volume of critically ill patients requiring your attention can suddenly increase. Thus, the NP may not expect or be prepared for these situations. Recognize when you begin to feel overwhelmed, intimidated, nervous, panicky, or things are spinning out of control. That is the exact moment you need to take a pause and ask for help. Access resources who can support you and your team.

Self-awareness and situational awareness are critical to being an excellent AG-ACNP. Self-awareness is the understanding when a situation is beyond your control. Situational awareness is the understanding of the knowledge, skills, and experience of those around you. Can they handle the situation? Are they doing the right things, in the right manner, in the right timeframe, or are they overwhelmed? Encourage them to ask for help from colleagues, the charge nurse, supervisors, and so forth. Timely access to resources is essential to support you, your team, and improve patient outcomes. Even experienced people still get these feelings, but the sign of an outstanding clinician is recognition of the situation and accessing additional resources.

KNOW YOUR RESOURCES

The second step is knowing who to call to ask for help. There are a variety of people you need to know for each shift. First is to know who your immediate backup is in the event of a patient decompensation. Additional resources you may need to access include

- the charge nurse,
- respiratory therapy,
- rapid-response team,
- airway management team,
- IV therapy team,
- trauma team, and
- other consultants

Immediate Backup

Of utmost importance is knowing who your immediate backup is, especially on night, weekend, and holiday shifts. Each institution, unit, and service is different and will have different people and different contact numbers. Take time early in your shift to see which senior resident, fellow, and attending are on call. Ensure you have their contact numbers (pager or cell phone) so you can reach each of them. This will save you time during an emergency. Recognize they may or may not be on campus, or may be tied up performing a procedure or in the operating room. They may need some lead time to join you at the bedside.

Fast Facts

Identify who your resources are, and write their names and contact info at the top of your handoff sheet for each shift. This expedites patient care when time matters.

Additional resources available to you include other clinicians and consultants. Nurse practitioners from your team as well as other services can serve as mentors and resources. Keep a list handy of clinicians and/or departments that are frequently consulted (see Table 2.1).

Table 2.1

Frequently Called Contacts

Contact	Phone or pager
Clinical	
Addiction medicine	
Anesthesia	
Cardiology	
Cardiothoracic surgery	
Colorectal surgery	
Dermatology	
Emergency department	
Endocrinology	
Infectious disease	
IV Team	
Gastroenterology	
Hematology/Oncology	
Hepatology	
Neurology	
Neurosurgery	
Ophthalmology	
Orthopedics	
Pain management	
Palliative care	
Physiatry	
Plastic surgery	
Psychiatry	
Pulmonary	
Radiology	
Surgery, General	
Transplant surgery	
Trauma	
Urology	

(*continued*)

Table 2.1

Frequently Called Contacts (*continued*)

Contact	Phone or pager
Vascular	
Other	
Departments	
Blood bank	
Case management	
Cath Lab	
CT Scan	
ECHO lab	
EEG	
Interventional radiology	
IV Team	
Laboratory	
Pastoral care	
Pharmacy	
Physical therapy	
Radiology	
Social work	
Ultrasound	
Vascular lab	
Other	
Administrative	
Administrative assistant	
Billing office	
Collaborating physician	
Employee health	
Manager	
Nurse manager	
Nursing supervisor	
Parking office	
Payroll	
Security	
Other	

Consultants

When calling a team to consult on your patient, call the team as early as possible in the shift. This courtesy allows them to prioritize their work and budget their time. To enhance efficiency, be sure to have the patient's name, medical record number, and room number ready. During the call:

1. State that you are calling them with a consult or to follow up on a previous consult.
2. Convey the urgency, clinical history/situation, and specific clinical question to be answered.
3. Provide your contact information for them to be able to reach you with any recommendations.
4. Finally, be sure to enter an actual order in the patient's chart so the consultant will be able to bill for their services.

WHEN TO "BUMP IT UP THE CHAIN"

Learning what needs to be escalated up the chain of command can be challenging. These can be either patient care situations, family concerns, or administrative issues. Some institutions have a list that require all providers, both NP and residents alike, to escalate specific patient-status changes to specific people. This list commonly includes:

- transfer from floor to step-down units or ICU
- unexpected intubations
- initiation of new vasopressors
- transfusion of more than two units of blood
- unplanned or emergent surgery or procedure
- cardiac arrest
- unexpected death
- admission and death without being seen by the attending physician

Some institutions require the resident or NP to staff the patient with an attending, who may be on call or available via a tele-ICU. Understanding the expectations and process up front can enhance patient outcomes and limit liabilities.

Fast Facts

When in doubt, make the call! Delaying communications when you are unclear on a diagnosis or treatment option commonly results in adverse consequences for the patient. Make the call!

Administrative Issues

Administrative issues such as patient safety concerns, compliance issues, harassment, or other negative behavior should be immediately reported to your supervisor. In addition, these should be in writing via incident reporting systems or minimally via email so they can be addressed in a timely fashion.

ATTENDING PREFERENCES

All attending physicians have their particular preferences or nuances. Learning these specifics initially can be challenging and can involve the school of hard knocks as you learn their preferences. Thus, it's helpful to ask senior residents, fellows, and other NPs on the team to give you an overview of specific attending preferences. Keep track of these items (mentally or write them in a pocket notebook) and you'll quickly look like a proficient NP. A few examples of provider preferences:

- the order in which patients are presented on rounds
- a focus on glycemic levels and control
- the precise surgery that was done
- culture results with day and duration of antibiotics
- specific enteral feeds with nutritional supplements and protein needs
- code status and legal medical decision-maker

These particulars commonly emerge through their lived experiences and have become important to them. Thus, by focusing on these details, we demonstrate respect for their values and priorities and will integrate ourselves into the team more efficiently.

Fast Facts

Keep track of attending physician preferences, and focus on customizing your presentations to ensure these points are covered.

Over time you will develop personal nuances too, such as updating diagnosis codes, minimizing lab draws, ordering/scheduling lab work at the same time to allow nurses to cluster care, cleaning up the order set to keep only current orders, and so forth.

In summary, learn who to call and how to access them in a timely fashion at the beginning of each shift. Identify key people who are oncall and can be readily available for backup should the need arise. Learn provider preferences early in your career, which will make your onboarding go more smoothly.

References

Green, B., Parry, D., Oeppen, R. S., Plint, S., Dale, T., & Brennan, P. A. (2017). Situational awareness—what it means for clinicians, its recognition and importance in patient safety. *Oral Diseases*, *23*(6), 721–725. https://doi.org/10.1111/odi.12547

Wright, M., & Endsley, M. (2008). Improving healthcare team communication: Building on lessons from aviation and aerospace. In *Building shared situation awareness in healthcare settings* (pp. 97–114). CRC Press. https://doi.org/10.1201/9781315588056-7

3

Admission, Discharge, Transfer

Hospitals are routinely at or exceeding capacity. With beds in high demand and emergency rooms overflowing, triaging, admitting and transferring patients to the appropriate level of care can be challenging. Understanding the institutional admission, discharge, and transfer criteria and processes is critical to ensuring appropriate utilization of resources and ensuring optimal patient outcomes.

In this chapter, you will learn

- criteria for appropriate placement of patients to intensive care, intermediate care, and ward care, with or without telemetry;
- considerations for triaging patients;
- options and criteria for post-hospital discharge facilities (long-term acute care hospital [LTACH], acute rehab, subacute rehab, skilled nursing facility [SNF], home healthcare, hospice);
- to identify the Centers for Medicare & Medicaid Services' (CMS) six conditions/procedures in the unplanned readmission measures.

ADMISSION, DISCHARGE, AND TRANSFER (ADT) CRITERIA

AG-ACNPs need to know the hospital's specific admission, discharge, and transfer (ADT) criteria and triage policies to match patient-specific needs while considering institutional resource limitations and therapeutic capabilities. Specifically, ICU admission decisions should be made based on patient-specific needs that can only be addressed in the ICU environment (see Tables 3.1 and 3.2). Consideration of life-supporting

Table 3.1

Types of Inpatients by Level of Care

Level & nursing ratio	Type of patients	Interventions
Intensive care 1:1 to 1:2	Critically ill patients who require care that can only be provided by specifically trained ICU staff that is not available elsewhere in the hospital, have clinical instability (e.g., status epilepticus, hypoxemia, and shock), are at high risk for imminent respiratory decline (e.g., impending intubation), or require hourly and/or invasive monitoring	Invasive interventions not provided elsewhere in the institution, such as CSF drainage for elevated ICP, invasive mechanical ventilation, vasopressors, ECMO, IABP, LVAD, or CRRT
Intermediate care ≤1:3	Unstable patients who need nursing interventions, laboratory workup and/or monitoring every 2–4 hours	Noninvasive ventilation, IV infusion or titration of vasodilators or antiarrhythmic agents
Telemetry ≤1:4	Stable patients who need close ECG monitoring for nonmalignant arrhythmias or laboratory work every 2–4 hours	IV infusion and titration of medications such as vasodilators or antiarrhythmics
General care ≤1:5	Stable patients who need testing and monitoring not more frequently than every 4 hours	IV antibiotics, IV chemotherapy, laboratory and/or radiologic workup

CRRT, continuous renal replacement therapy; CSF, cerebrospinal fluid; ECMO, extracorporeal membrane oxygenation; IABP, intra-aortic balloon pump; ICP, intracranial pressure; LVAD, left ventricular assist device.

therapies; available clinical expertise; prioritization according to the patient's condition; diagnoses; bed availability; objective parameters such as vital signs; laboratory values; potential for the patient to benefit from interventions; and prognosis.

Tips for Triaging ICU Level of Care

- Patients should be admitted or discharged based on potential to benefit from ICU care.
- Triage decisions should be made without bias. Age, race, ethnicity, social status, gender, sexual identity, preference, and finances should never be considered in triage decisions.
- Overtriage is more acceptable and preferable to undertriaging patients.
- Critically ill patients should be transferred from the ED to the ICU within 6 hours.

Table 3.2

Prioritizing ICU Patients

Level of care	Priority	Type of patient
ICU	1	Critically ill patients who require life support for organ failure, intensive monitoring, and therapies only provided in the ICU environment. Life support includes invasive ventilation, CRRT, invasive hemodynamic monitoring to direct aggressive hemodynamic interventions, ECMO, IABP, and other situations requiring critical care (e.g., patients with severe hypoxemia or in shock).
ICU	2	Priority-one patients with significantly lower probability of recovery and who would like to receive intensive care therapies but no CPR (e.g., patients with metastatic cancer and respiratory failure secondary to pneumonia or in septic shock requiring vasopressors).
IMCU	3	Patients with organ dysfunction who require intensive monitoring and/or therapies (i.e., NIV), or who could be managed at a level of care less than ICU (e.g., postop patients who need close monitoring for risk of deterioration, i.e., respiratory insufficiency with intermittent noninvasive ventilation). These patients could need ICU care if early management fails to prevent deterioration or there is no IMCU level of care within the hospital.
IMCU	4	Patients as above but with less probability of recovery/survival (e.g., patients with underlying metastatic disease) who do not want to be intubated or resuscitated. If the hospital does not have an IMCU, these patients could be considered for ICU.
Palliative	5	Terminal or moribund patients with no possibility of recovery; such patients, in general, are not appropriate for ICU (unless they are potential organ donors). In cases where individuals have clearly declined ICU therapies or have irreversible processes, palliative care should be offered.

CPR, cardiopulmonary resuscitation; CRRT, continuous renal replacement therapy; ECMO, extracorporeal membrane oxygenation; IABP, intra-aortic balloon pump; IMCU, intermediate care unit; NIV, noninvasive ventilation.

- Considering the frequent lack of readily available ICU beds, all AG-ACNPs should be prepared to deliver critical care at the patient's current location.
- Patients with risk factors to decompensate should be monitored closely and managed in a higher level of care than a ward in the immediate postoperative period.
- Base decisions to admit an older adult (>80 years) patient to ICU on the patient's comorbidities, severity of illness, prehospital functional

Chapter 3 Admission, Discharge, Transfer

status, patient preferences with regard to life-sustaining treatment, and likelihood to benefit from the intervention/escalation of level of care.

- ICU admission of cancer patients should be decided based on the same criteria established for all critically ill patients, with careful consideration of their long-term prognosis.
- Reassess ICU interventions for all critically ill patients, especially those with advanced cancer, and discuss life-sustaining interventions with the patient and legal decision-maker.

Discharge from ICU

- Discharge a patient from the ICU to a lower acuity area when a patient's physiologic status has stabilized and the need for ICU monitoring and treatment is resolved.
- Discharge parameters should be based on ICU admission criteria, the admitting criteria for the next lower level of care, institutional availability of these resources, patient prognosis, physiologic stability, and ongoing active interventions.
- When able, avoid discharging patients from ICU "after hours" ("night shift" or after 7 p.m.).
- Discharge patients at high risk for mortality and readmission (high severity of illness, multiple comorbidities, physiologic instability, ongoing organ support) to a step-down unit or long-term acute care hospital as opposed to the regular ward.
- Standardize processes (written and oral) for both provider and nursing processes when discharging from ICU to reduce risk of readmission.

LEVELS OF CARE POSTDISCHARGE

Discharge planning is an essential element of an AG-ACNP's role (see Table 3.3). Collaboration with the case manager is essential to ensure patients are discharged to the appropriate level of care. AG-ACNPs need to possess knowledge of the patient needs and expectations of the postdischarge settings. Discharge options include home without services, home with homecare or outpatient services, acute inpatient rehabilitation, LTACHs, subacute rehabilitation, SNFs, and hospice.

READMISSIONS

The CMS includes six conditions/procedures in the unplanned readmission measures in the hospital readmissions reduction program. This is a pay-for-performance program that reduces payments to hospitals with

Table 3.3

Post–Acute Care Discharge Options for Inpatient Rehabilitation

	Subacute rehabilitation	Acute rehabilitation	LTACH
Type of care provided	Skilled nursing or skilled rehabilitation services for the short term on a daily basis in an inpatient setting after an inpatient stay of 3 or more days	Intensive rehabilitation therapy in an inpatient hospital environment. Patient requires and is expected to benefit from 3 hours or more of therapy, 5 days per week	Continued hospital level of care
Typical medical conditions	Heart failure; hip and femur procedures; joint replacement; kidney and urinary tract infections, infections	Brain injury; lower extremity fracture; major joint replacements; neurological disorders, stroke	Complex medical conditions; complex wound/burn management; mechanical ventilation weaning
Daily therapy requirements	1–1.5 hours	>3 hours	NA
Average length of stay	27 days	13.1 days	26.6 days
Average cost for care per patient	$10,800	$17,100	$38,500

LTACH, long-term acute care hospital.

excess readmissions. The publicly reported 30-day risk-standardized unplanned readmission measures include:

- acute myocardial infarction (AMI)
- chronic obstructive pulmonary disease (COPD)
- heart failure (HF)
- pneumonia
- coronary artery bypass graft (CABG) surgery
- elective primary total hip and/or total knee arthroplasty (THA/TKA)

AG-ACNPs play a vital role in preventing hospital readmissions. NPs are commonly called upon to lead teams to reduce readmissions. Resources for NPs to aid in reducing readmissions include the AHRQ RED toolkit: https://www.ahrq.gov/patient-safety/settings/hospital/red/toolkit/index.html.

Learn about your hospital's readmission rates. Identify ways you can make an impact. Engage with departmental committees. NPs can make a huge impact!

In summary, AG-ACNPs must know the institutional capacity and capabilities as a whole and of each individual unit. This includes the skills, knowledge, and experience of nurses and other staff, number of beds, and the criteria for admission, transfer, and discharge to and from these units. Knowledge of discharge requirements and facility capabilities can aid in efficient patient discharges to appropriate facilities. Be aware of your hospital readmission rates, and advocate to mobilize resources to safely discharge patients to the most appropriate levels of care.

References

Agency for Healthcare Research and Quality. (2020). *Re-Engineered Discharge (RED) toolkit*. www.ahrq.gov/patient-safety/settings/hospital/red/toolkit/index.html

CMS. (2021). *Re-admission measures*. www.qualitynet.org/inpatient/measures/readmission

Nates, J. L., Nunnally, M., Kleinpell, R., Blosser, S., Goldner, J., Birriel, B., Fowler, C. S., Byrum, D., Miles, W. S., Bailey, H., & Sprung, C. L. (2016). ICU admission, discharge, and triage guidelines: A framework to enhance clinical operations, development of institutional policies, and further research. *Critical Care Medicine*, *44*(8), 1553–1602. https://doi.org/10.1097/ccm.0000000000001856

Stefanacci, R. (2015). Admission criteria for facility-based post-acute services. *Ann Long-Term Care Clinical Care Aging*, *23*, 18–20.

4

Documentation

Documenting completely and thoroughly is essential to providing high-quality, comprehensive patient care. In nursing, if "it's not documented, it's not done." In the nurse practitioner world, if it's not documented, the hospital and/or group practice won't be paid for the higher level of acuity and care that is provided. Thus, failure to document will also have a financial and potentially legal impact.

In this chapter, you will learn

- key elements of documentation all AG-ACNPs must know;
- elements of a thorough history and physical;
- to identify the common best practices to review on every patient, every day;
- fundamentals of admission orders;
- to discuss components of a discharge summary; and
- to identify core components of death pronouncement documentation.

HISTORY AND PHYSICAL

The history and physical (H&P) is much more than just taking a history and performing a physical exam. A comprehensive H&P also includes stating the primary diagnosis, consideration of differential diagnoses, overall assessment of the patient's admitting diagnosis, any complications and concomitant conditions, as well as the treatment plan and billing language. The H&P should also address pertinent past medical history problems, including continued management of or adjustments to each.

History of Present Illness (HPI)

The HPI describes the status of the current illness. Two commonly used acronyms to explore symptoms are OLDCAART or the seven cardinal features:

- OLDCAART: Onset, location, duration, character, aggravating factors, alleviating factors, radiation, timing
- seven cardinal features: temporal characteristics, location, intensity, quality, aggravating and alleviating factors, related symptoms

Past Medical History (PMH)

- diagnoses that are in old medical records if they still apply
- new diagnoses that may not be in the chart but which are verifiable

Past Surgical History (PSH)

- all surgeries
- includes procedures such as cardiac catheterizations, colonoscopies, and so forth

Allergies

- includes medications, environmental, foods, IV contrast, and so forth

Medications

- prescribed medications
- over-the-counter medications
- herbals and supplements
- anything borrowed from others or bought on the street

Social History (SH)

- employment, both current and previous jobs
- service in the armed forces; if so, any exposures or injuries, residual effects/deficits, and PTSD
- living arrangements and use of assistive devices
- ever smoked, if so, how much, for how long
- alcohol consumption with quantification and illicit substances
- stress, including financial stress
- being caregiver for others
- religion and other support mechanisms

Family History (FH)

- mother, father, siblings, children, aunts/uncles, grandparents

Review of Systems (ROS)

- a series of questions, organized by organ system, to identify organ dysfunction and disease (see Table 4.1).

Table 4.1

Common ROS Questions	
Constitutional	Fever, chills, fatigue, anorexia, weight gain or loss
HEENT	Change in vision, eye pain, double vision, flashing lights, last eye exam, glaucoma or cataracts, sore throat, congestion, sinus trouble, hay fever, epistaxis, hoarse voice, dental problems, bleeding gums
Neck	Neck pain or stiffness, swollen glands, lumps
Cardiovascular	Chest pain, pain on exertion or stress, palpitations, racing heart, lightheadedness, heart murmur, weight gain, blood clots, swelling in hands or feet/legs, blue fingers/toes, pain in legs with ambulation
Respiratory	Shortness of breath, exertional dyspnea, paroxysmal nocturnal dyspnea, wheezing, cough (if so, is it productive, and if so, what color?)
Abdominal	Abdominal pain, nausea, vomiting, change in stools, constipation, diarrhea, last normal BM, heartburn or belching, food intolerance, pain after eating, rectal bleeding
Genitourinary	Difficulty urinating, pain or burning on urination, nocturia, urgency, incontinence, decreased urine stream, blood in urine, enlarged prostate
Hematology	Easy bruising, bleeding, previous transfusions
Immune	Recent sick contacts, recent illnesses, recent hospitalizations, recent antibiotics or immunizations, night sweats
Endocrine	Increased thirst, increased urine production, heat or cold intolerance, excessive sweating
Musculoskeletal	Muscle pain, bone pain, joint pain, weakness, muscle cramping, cramping with walking, balance difficulties, difficulty with coordination
Integumentary	Rashes, wounds, itching, change in hair or nails, jaundice
Neurological	Headaches, head injury, seizures, loss of consciousness, fainting, tremors, involuntary movements, numbness, dizziness
Psychiatric	Anxiety, depression, suicidal ideation, memory problems, insomnia, change in mood

HEENT, head, eyes, ears, nose, and throat.

Physical Exam

- At least two bullet points per body system, including:
  - general, HEENT, neurological, respiratory, cardiovascular, abdominal, genitourinary, musculoskeletal, integumentary.

Assessment

- A statement summarizing the reason for admission and current status of the admitting diagnosis.
- Include any complicating factors or conditions.

Plan

- Can be problem focused, for straight-forward healthy patients.
- By body system, for more medically complex patients.
- Or for critically ill multi-organ-system patients, can be organized by individual problems within each body system.

Diagnoses

- Precision matters when documenting problems. Comprehensive and detailed problem lists are essential to good patient care (see Table 4.2). Using ICD-10 diagnoses is important. Be sure to avoid slang terminology. Coding and billing specialists are not trained clinicians who can interpret abbreviations or acronyms. Common terminology to be familiar with:
  - Principal diagnosis: The condition established after workup is completed and is chiefly responsible for admission to the hospital. If this is not readily known, list the differential diagnoses or articulate a "working diagnosis" if further diagnostics are pending.
  - Secondary diagnoses: All conditions that coexist at the time of admission, develop during the admission, or continue to affect the patient during the current hospitalization. These are any conditions that require assessment, evaluation, monitoring, or treatment.
  - Present on admission: Documenting healthcare-associated infections (HAI) that exist at the time of admission is critical. These HAIs include, but are not limited to, pressure ulcers and respective stages, central line–associated bloodstream infections (CLABSI), catheter-associated urinary tract infection (CAUTI), and ventilator-associated pneumonia (VAP). Failure to document these conditions as present on admission could cause liability for such events to fall within the hospitalization and adversely impact quality reporting and finances for the institution.

Table 4.2

Examples of Recommended Terminology and Terms to Avoid		
Body system	**Recommend**	**Avoid**
Neurologic	Encephalopathy Hemiparesis Epilepsy Intellectual disability	Altered mental status Left- or right-sided weakness Seizure disorder Global developmental delay
Respiratory	Acute/chronic respiratory failure Bronchopulmonary dysplasia Pulmonary edema	Acute/chronic respiratory insufficiency Chronic lung disease Lungs wet, diuresis
Cardiovascular	Shock (septic, cardiogenic, etc.)	Low blood pressure on pressors
Renal	Acute kidney injury or failure Chronic kidney disease with stage Hypokalemia	Acute renal insufficiency Chronic kidney disease (without stage) Low potassium or replete K
Gastrointestinal	Malnutrition Dysphagia	Underweight or low BMI Aspiration, gastrostomy-dependence
Hematology	Anemia Pancytopenia secondary to chemotherapy Coagulopathy	Low hemoglobin List only transfusion parameters Elevated INR
Infectious disease	Sepsis, severe sepsis, septic shock Septic shock secondary to UTI Pneumonia (with type/organism)	SIRS/Sepsis physiology Urosepsis Consolidation on CXR
Endocrine	Adrenal insufficiency	Document only stress dose steroids

BMI, body mass index; CXR, chest X-ray; INR, international normalized ratio; SIRS, systemic inflammatory response syndrome; UTI, urinary tract infection.

Billing Time and Codes

- Billing time and codes should be included at the bottom of each note.
- Include a summary statement indicating the specific need for the level of care and the specific interventions that require that level of care (e.g., "This patient is critically ill due to acute hypoxemic and hypercarbic respiratory failure, requiring multiple mechanical ventilation adjustments.")

DAILY PROGRESS NOTES

For a member of a primary team responsible for the holistic care of the patient, daily progress notes are required. To fulfill billing requirements, key elements of the daily progress note include

- the reason the patient remains hospitalized or requires ICU level of care;
- summary of 24-hour events;
- current exam;
- current, pertinent laboratory data;
- current X-ray findings; and
- assessment and plan for primary problem and all problems actively being managed.

Many institutions also include a section in each daily progress note entitled *best practices* or *global issues checklist* to review common concepts among all ICU patients.

BEST PRACTICES

Several areas should be addressed on a daily basis. These can be addressed within each system of the note or addressed at the end of the note:

- Pain.
  - Identify the current status of the patient's pain and analgesic regimen and pain-scale goals.
- Sedation.
  - Identify the goal Richmond Agitation Sedation Scale (RASS) or Riker Sedation-Agitation Scale (RIKERS) score and current sedation regimen.
  - Note any sedation holiday or awakening trial, or document contraindications to sedation holiday/sedation vacation/ spontaneous awakening trial.
- Delirium assessment and treatment.
- Evaluate culture results daily, and evaluate for de-escalation of antibiotics.
- Identify current intravascular fluid balance status (hypo, hyper, or euvolemic), and set a goal for the next 24 hours.
- Foley.
  - Document insertion date, location placed or date changed, and determine if still needed.
- Invasive lines.
  - Document date inserted, whether or not they are still needed, and for what reason.
- Glycemic control.
  - Are blood sugars within goal, state goal finger stick blood sugar (FSBS), and document the current regimen.

- DVT prophylaxis.
    - Document mechanical and chemoprophylaxis or any contraindications to either; if contraindicated, state why and when expected to be able to initiate or seek an alternative, such as an IVC filter.
- Stress ulcer prophylaxis.
    - Document indication and treatment. Evaluate if it can be discontinued, or note if it is a home medication, so as not to inadvertently discontinue.
- Document current code status and any plans to address with the patient or family.
- Patient's decision-making capacity.
    - Does the patient have capacity today?
- Medical decision-maker.
    - If patient does not have capacity, who is the legal decision-maker?
    - What is the best number to reach them?
- Family updates.
    - Who and what topics did you update?

ORDERING AND PRESCRIBING

Admission orders need to be complete and match your plan of care as outlined in the H&P. Many AG-ACNPs will write an initial order to admit once the decision to admit has been determined. Writing this initial admit order helps expedite the process to get the patient a bed and get them out of the emergency department. Subsequently, as the H&P is developed, the AG-ACNP will write any remaining orders. An easy mnemonic to ensure complete admission orders is entered to remember the ABCs as follows:

General Admission Orders

- A—Admit to or transfer to – need to list specific attending and service
- A—Allergies with reaction
- A—Activity and any limitations or restrictions
    - Weight-bearing status
    - Head of bed elevation
- B—Because—what is the admitting diagnosis?
- C—Condition—critical, stable, and so forth per hospital guidelines
- C—Code status and vital signs (VS) (specify to include O2 saturation, neuro and/or vascular checks)
- D—Disability – any special spinal precautions, assistive devices, and so forth
- D—Diet, or Nothing by mouth (NPO)

- D—DVT prophylaxis, sequential compression devices or foot pumps
- E—Electrolyte replacements
- F—Fluids, continuous-maintenance IV fluids or boluses
- F—Foley insertion
- G—Gastric tubes: orogastric tube (OGT), nasogastric tube (NGT), gastric tube (GT), small bore feeding tubes, and so forth
- G—Glucose monitoring
- I—Incentive Spirometer
- N—Nursing care
- Notifications – for example: "Call the Advanced Practice Registered Nurse for … "
  - Identify specific vital signs and customize to each patient.
  - Any patient-specific criteria – neurological changes, vascular changes, and so forth
- O—O2, noninvasive ventilation or ventilator settings
- Provider consultations
  - Must write an order for them to actually bill for services.
  - Include reason or clinical question they should answer.
  - Be sure to call them yourself to request consultation.
- Tubes/lines/drains, what and where they are, and what should be done with them
- Wound management and dressings

Medication Orders

- Perform medication reconciliation
  - Review each medication and elect to continue or discontinue each item.
  - Document a diagnosis and reason decision to continue or hold each individual medication.
  - Review home medication list daily to evaluate if medications can be restarted or continue to hold.
- GI stress ulcer prophylaxis—indications:
  - Concurrent administration of glucocorticoids.
  - Intubated for >48 hours.
  - Active GI bleeding.
  - Recent head or spinal cord injury.
  - Consider H2 blockers first, then proton pump inhibitors.
- Bowel management regimen
- DVT prophylaxis
  - Refer to VTE guidelines.
  - Document any contraindications.
- Glucose management regimen
- PRN medications
  - Pain regimen
  - Antiemetic
  - Constipation

Diagnostic Testing

- Order any additional workup needed to make or clarify a diagnosis.
- Serial laboratory testing (troponins, CBCs, etc.)
- Decide upon which labs you need in the morning (e.g., BMP, magnesium).
- Diagnostic studies:
  - When ordering diagnostic tests, list specific patient signs and symptoms to answer a clinical question.
  - <u>Always</u> write an indication (symptom) for test (e.g., fever, chest pain (CP), headache (HA), abdominal (ABD) pain, edema, shortness of breath).
  - Do <u>not</u> write the suspected diagnosis.
    - RIGHT: CXR for shortness of breath
    - WRONG: rule out (R/O) … (i.e., R/O pneumonia) as the indication
  - Add a comment to the order to guide the interpreting provider indicating the clinical question that needs to be answered (e.g., computed tomography (CT) abdomen/pelvis with contrast for fever. Please evaluate left lower quadrant (LLQ) for abscess or anastamotic leak, as patient had sigmoid resection 7 days ago).
  - Take time to discuss the exam that is needed to ensure the clinical question is answered with the most appropriate diagnostic test for the particular patient given their current clinical condition.
- CT scans and magnetic resonance imaging (MRI) scans:
  - Discuss with team whether contrast is needed.
    - Need for oral (PO), IV, or per rectum (PR) contrast
    - Abdominal abscesses: need both IV and PO contrast
    - PR contrast is used to evaluate for colonic perforation or anastomosis leakage.
    - To identify an arterial occlusion, IV contrast in the arterial phase is required.
    - Contrast is not needed to evaluate the pleural space.
    - If in doubt, call the radiologist to discuss the clinical question to answer, and request their recommendations.
  - Determine phase of contrast.
    - Arterial phase highlights arteries/arterial blood flow.
    - Intraparenchymal—highlights the organs.
    - Venous phase shows veins and venous outflow obstructions.
  - Concern for contrast-induced nephropathy.
    - Creatinine limit ~ 1.5.
    - Hydrate with NS IV to protect kidneys.
    - Consider alternative diagnostic test.

Choosing Wisely® Campaign

The Choosing Wisely campaign seeks to apply evidence to reduce unnecessary testing and interventions to contain escalating healthcare costs without causing harm. NPs should decide on a daily basis whether testing or interventions are essential to patient care. Consider whether the additional information will change the management plan or make an additional diagnosis that could require additional treatments. The Choosing Wisely campaign has partnered with the various specialty societies to develop a list of recommendations for each specialty. The following recommendations apply to the critical care and hospital medicine teams:

- Don't order diagnostic tests at regular intervals (such as every day), but rather in response to specific clinical questions.
- Don't transfuse red blood cells as the sole intervention for expansion of circulatory volume unless deemed necessary for patients experiencing severe hemorrhage.
- Don't transfuse red blood cells in hemodynamically stable, nonbleeding ICU patients with a hemoglobin concentration greater than 7 g/dL.
- Don't use parenteral nutrition in adequately nourished critically ill patients within the first 7 days of an ICU stay.
- Don't deeply sedate mechanically ventilated patients without a specific indication and without daily attempts to lighten sedation.
- Don't continue life support for patients at high risk for death or severely impaired functional recovery without offering patients and their families the alternative of care focused entirely on comfort.
- Don't place, or leave in place, urinary catheters for incontinence or convenience or monitoring of output for patients who are not critically ill (acceptable indications: critical illness, obstruction, hospice, perioperatively for <2 days for urologic procedures; use weights instead to monitor diuresis).
- Don't prescribe medications for stress ulcer prophylaxis to medical inpatients unless at high risk for GI complications.
- Don't order continuous telemetry monitoring outside of the ICU without using a protocol that governs continuation.

Fast Facts

Will ordering a diagnostic test change the management plan or make an additional diagnosis that requires additional treatments? If the answer is no, then do not order the test or spend the money.

PROCEDURAL NOTES

Having secured informed consent (see Chapter 20, Ethical and Legal Issues, for details of the informed consent process) and immediately upon completion of a procedure, thorough documentation of the procedure is required. When documenting a clinical procedure, important elements include:

- that a timeout was performed; include the time and persons present
- the procedure that was performed
- reason procedure was performed (e.g., for vasopressor support, respiratory failure)
- the patient's side and site procedure was performed
- type and size of line or tube inserted
- technique used
- use of any device to guide insertion (e.g., ultrasound, glide scope)
- any images obtained
- return or flow of blood or other bodily fluids, as well as color and amount of fluid
- specimens sent for analysis
- how the patient tolerated the procedure
- any medications used during the procedure, such as lidocaine or conscious sedation
- results of any diagnostics to confirm placement of tubes, lines, or drains

DEATH PRONOUNCEMENT NOTE

When a patient expires in the hospital, a separate note pronouncing the death is required in addition to a discharge summary. This note contains a physical examination and notation of time of death. Notification of family, the attending physician, surgical teams, and any consulting services, as well as institutional admitting office, is expected. Additional notification of the patient's primary care provider (PCP) is good practice. The following is a sample pronouncement note:

I was called to the patient's bedside to pronounce that the patient (insert name) had died. No spontaneous movements were noted. There was no response to verbal or noxious tactile stimuli. Pupils were fixed and dilated. Auscultated for heart and lung sound and observed for chest movement for 2 minutes. No heart or lung sounds were present. No chest movements were observed. Carotid artery was palpated, and no pulse was appreciated. Time of death was (insert time). The family was present (or notified) of the time of death. Dr. (insert attending name) was notified of death.

Be sure to review the cause of death with the attending of record. DO NOT write "cardiopulmonary arrest" as the immediate cause of death. Identify what caused the cardiopulmonary arrest.

DISCHARGE SUMMARY

A discharge summary contains three main sections, a brief overview, details of the hospital stay, and detailed discharge instructions and recommendations. Each of these sections has additional details that should be included (see Table 4.3). Many of these elements are automatically imported from the electronic medical record.

Table 4.3

Elements of a Discharge Summary	
Brief overview	Brief summary of reason for hospital stay
	Admitting/discharging providers
	PCP at discharge and contact info
	Admission/discharge date
	Primary and secondary diagnoses
	Discharge disposition and location
	Guardian/POA contact information
	Code status
	Active issues requiring follow-up
	Medication-monitoring instructions
	Scheduled follow-up appointments
	Recommended labs/imaging or other procedures to be done after discharge
	Test results pending at time of discharge
Details of hospital stay	Presenting problem/history of present illness
	Hospital course
	Operative and other procedures performed
	Consults
	Pertinent laboratory results
	Pathology results
	Physical exam at time of discharge, including vital signs and weight
	Cognitive status at discharge
Detailed discharge instructions	Diet orders
	Fall risk status
	Activity orders
	Wound-care instructions
	Bowel/bladder management/care
	Patient care instructions—that is, reasons to call or return to be seen and specialty-specific recommendations
	Patient's goals/preferences
	Discharge medications
	Contact information for discharging provider
	Author of discharge summary

PCP, primary care provider; POA, power of attorney.

The brief summary should be a high-level summary, not a day-by-day reiteration. Rather, it should state the diagnosis, causative agent, treatments, current status of the problem, and any ongoing treatments or future plans. This summary can be outlined in either a problem-based or system-based approach, or for medically complex patients can be done by problem within each system.

Fast Facts

The brief overview of a discharge summary should be a high-level summary of the hospital stay.

Documentation Pearls

- Document all diagnoses associated with a patient, including secondary diagnoses, to accurately reflect the patients' overall condition.
- Support diagnoses with clinical assessment and data.
- Identify the underlying etiology causing the diagnosis.
- Clarify the status of each diagnosis as acute, subacute, chronic (e.g., acute on chronic hypercarbic respiratory failure).
- Provide additional details on diagnoses.
  - the type, stage, and laterality of the diagnosis (e.g., chronic kidney disease (CKD) stage III, right hemiparesis, type 1 diabetes mellitus)
- Make connections between conditions (e.g., septic shock d/t urinary tract infection (UTI) complicated by acute kidney injury).
- When unknown, use terms such as "possible," "probable," "likely," or "suspected."
- Documentation of active disease processes should be continued daily through the admission and included in the discharge summary.
- Update conditions daily as they evolve. Options include "improving," "worsening," "stable," or "resolved."
- Use caution with the copy-and-paste functionality of the electronic medical record. This functionality leaves room for ongoing documentation errors (e.g., "patient extubated today" being documented for four consecutive days).
- Avoid prohibited abbreviations. The joint commission's list of "Do not use" abbreviations includes those found in Table 4.4.

In summary, thorough documentation is crucial to patient care, can impact financial revenue, and protect in medical-legal scenarios. Take time to become familiar with coding and billing staff. Answer clinical documentation queries promptly so billing can be detailed, accurate, and at the highest level to facilitate the highest reimbursement.

Table 4.4

Prohibited Abbreviations

Avoid:	Rationale	Instead write:
U or u	Can be mistaken for 0, 4, or mL	Units
IU	Can be mistaken for IV or 10	International units
Q.D., QD, q.d., qd, Q.O.D., QOD, q.o.d., qod	Mistaken for each other	Daily Every other day
Trailing zero, .0 Lacks leading zero, .X mg	Decimal point is missed	X mg 0.X mg
MS MSO4 or MgSO4	Confused with one another	Morphine Morphine or magnesium sulfate
> for greater than < for less than	Misinterpreted as seven or L or confused with each other	Greater than Less than
Abbreviations for drug names	Can be confused with other drugs or similar abbreviations	Write out full drug name
Apothecary units	Unfamiliar to many providers Confused with metric units	Use metric units
@	Confused with 2	at
mL	Can be confused with u	mL, milligram, mL (mL preferred)
ug	Mistaken for milligram and results in 1,000-fold overdose	mcg, microgram

References

Choosing Wisely. *ABIM Foundation*. www.choosingwisely.org/clinician-lists/

Dean, S. M., Gilmore-Bykovskyi, A., Buchanan, J., Ehlenfeldt, B., & Kind, A. J. (2016). Design and hospital-wide implementation of a standardized discharge summary in an electronic health record. *The Joint Commission Journal on Quality and Patient Safety, 42*(11).

Official "Do Not Use" List. (2019). www.jointcommission.org/-/media/tjc/documents/resources/patient-safety-topics/do_not_use_list_6_28_19.pdf

Sanderson, A. L., & Burns, J. P. (2020). Clinical Documentation for intensivists: The impact of diagnosis documentation. *Critical Care Medicine, 48*(4), 579–587.

5

Coding and Billing

Comprehensive and detailed documentation defines the higher level of acuity seen in hospitalized patients. Documenting completely and thoroughly, including a complete list of active problems and comorbidities, is essential to provide good patient care. The institution relies on clinician documentation to ensure the hospital is reimbursed by the level of acuity, thus better documentation yields higher reimbursement. The documentation MUST support the billing claims.

In this chapter, you will learn

- to differentiate between hospital and group practice billing,
- the required components of evaluation and management (E&M) codes,
- to differentiate between CPT codes and ICD-10 codes,
- to identify the components that compromise initial and subsequent care billing, and
- the elements for critical care billing.

Hospital Versus Group Practice Billing

When discussing coding and billing, it's important to recognize there are different codes for hospitals and group practices. Hospitals bill insurance for the care of the patients whose diagnoses are coded into diagnosis-related groups (DRGs). These are the codes for the medical diagnoses that NPs manage. Hospitals can also bill for the technical component of many procedures. This includes the space, technology and overhead to perform procedures,such as cardiac catheterizations

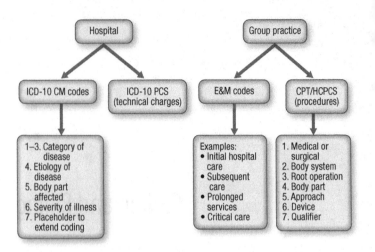

Figure 5.1 Overview of hospital and group practice coding.

and operations, and so forth. Procedures are denoted by the procedural classification system (PCS) for hospital billing. Group practices bill for providers' professional services. Professional billing is determined by the codes found in the Current Procedural Terminology (CPT) codebook and the Healthcare Common Procedure Coding System (HCPCS) book. These codebooks have all codes related to providers performing procedures and E&M codes which are used for admissions, critical care, daily care and discharges, consultations, and others (see Figure 5.1).

One of the most critical pieces of information for NPs to know is whether they were hired to bill professionally or to solely support various departments in the hospital only. If you aren't sure, you need to ask, because only NPs whose work is reimbursed by a group practice can bill for their professional services. Many hospitals do hire NPs to directly provide support to surgeons, freeing up the surgeon to operate more or see more new patients, which maximizes productivity and reimbursement. The cost of pre- and postoperative care is included in a 90-day global period, thus services related to surgery cannot be billed during the global period surrounding the surgery.

Fast Facts

In order for an NP to bill for services, the NP needs to know whether they were hired as an employee of the hospital or group practice. The hiring manager will be able to answer this question. NPs can only bill for professional services if their services are billed by a group practice.

ICD-10 CM Codes

The International Classification of Diseases, 10th Revision (ICD) clinical modifications codes are a series of alphanumeric coding to describe a disease state. In short, these codes represent patient diagnoses and problems. These codes are used for professional billing and hospital billing. A simplified sample demonstrates the formatting of the coding:

A01—{Disease}

- A01.0 {Disease} of the lungs
  - A01.01 ... simple
  - A01.02 ... complex
- A01.020 ... affecting the trachea
- A01.021 ... affecting the cardiopulmonary system
  - A01.021A ... initial encounter
  - A01.021D ... subsequent encounter
  - A01.021S ... sequela

These codes are commonly built directly into electronic medical records. The NP is responsible to build and maintain an accurate problem list and specify these details in the assessment and plan portion of the notes. Hospital coding specialists will routinely request additional or clarifying data to enhance the specificity. Be sure to respond promptly to these queries.

Diagnosis-Related Groups

The ICD-10 codes from an admission encounter are compiled and assigned into a DRG of similar conditions that consume comparative hospital resources and length of stay. DRGs take into consideration the illness severity, comorbid conditions, and mortality risk to calculate reimbursement.

Case Mix Index

The case mix index (CMI) measures the severity of illness or complexity of the inpatient population. The calculation is an average of the relative weights of all DRGs of a hospital over time periods. The higher the case mix index, the more complex the hospital population with higher acuity levels and greater utilization of resources. Provider documentation of comorbid conditions and complications drives up the case mix index. Case mix index is linked to hospital payments. Thus, accuracy and completeness of documentation translates into higher hospital reimbursement.

Hospital reimbursement is critical, as many hospitals contract with group practices for services, such as critical care services. The hospital pays the group practice, which in turn allows the group practice to pay their employees, including NP salaries. Thus, to ensure NP salaries are covered, it is imperative that NPs provide exemplary documentation in the medical records to drive up the DRG and the CMI.

Technical Charges

Hospitals can also bill for technical charges, which are charges for the use of the hospital facilities. Technical charges include overhead, room and board, nursing care, equipment, and so forth. Examples include the technical component of performing a heart catheterization. The physician would bill for his skill of performing and interpreting the procedure, whereas the hospital would bill the technical charge for the cath lab room; equipment, including fluoroscopy and catheters; nurses; technicians; and so forth for the procedure.

Healthcare Common Procedure Coding System (HCPCS)

The HCPCS coding system is a national system of codes for medical providers to submit billing claims for healthcare services to Medicare and other insurance companies in a consistent method. HCPCS is comprised of two sets of codes: HCPCS Level I and HCPCS Level II. HCPCS Level I codes are the current procedural terminology (CPT) codes used to submit claims to payers for services and procedures performed by providers, hospitals, clinics, and laboratories. HCPCS Level II codes are the procedure codes set for providers and medical equipment suppliers for medical devices, supplies, medications, transportation services, and so forth. In the following sections we discuss HCPCS Level I codes for procedures and E&M services commonly used by AG-ACNPs.

ICD-10 Procedure Coding System (PCS) Codes

ICD-10 PCS codes are the codes used by providers to bill for procedures (see Exhibit 5.1). Common bedside procedures performed by AG-ACNPs include suturing, central venous catheter insertion, arterial line insertion, paracentesis, thoracentesis, intubations, chest tube insertions, and so forth.

Exhibit 5.1 Components of ICD-10 PCS codes:

- Section relates to type of procedure.
- Body system
- Root operation specified objective of the procedure.
- Body part—specific body part/system on which procedure is performed.
- Approach is the technique used to reach the site of the procedure.
- Device specifies any devices that remain after the procedure has been completed.
- Qualifier provides additional information about the procedure.

E&M codes are the codes used by providers to bill insurance companies for their professional services to diagnose and treat patient conditions. Inpatient NPs commonly bill for observation care, initial hospital care, subsequent hospital care, consultations, critical care time, prolonged services, and discharges.

Inpatient Admission Versus Observation Status

The severity of the patient's illness and the intensity of services provided need to justify an acute hospital level of care. To qualify for inpatient status, the provider should expect the patient to require hospital care that spans at least two midnights. While AG-ANCPs can perform the admission process, the Centers for Medicare and Medicaid Services (CMS) requires a physician to certify that inpatient hospital services were reasonable and necessary. Medical necessity for inpatient care is determined by assessment of the patient's history and physical (H&P) and patient-specific risk factors at the time of admission.

Observation status is considered an outpatient status, which represents a set of clinically appropriate short-term services. Observation requires ONE of the following:

- diagnostic evaluation (e.g., rule out MI)
- acute treatment and evaluation of this treatment (e.g., observe for drug reaction)
- monitoring for event (e.g., arrhythmia)
- recovery (e.g., from drug/alcohol ingestion)

Once deemed observation, further data from the assessment, treatment, or reassessment will guide the decision whether patients require ongoing treatment with full admission or will be able to be discharged. This determination can frequently be made within the first 24 hours; however, it can be made within up to 48 hours and still qualify as observation. At the 48 hours, the determination to discharge or admit to inpatient must be made. This is informally known as the "two-midnight rule." A patient who stays beyond two midnights and clinically continues to require hospital level of care qualifies for inpatient admission.

Specific E&M Codes

The documentation requirements for both observation and inpatient care do not differ significantly. There are four main elements needed to bill for specific E&M codes, which include history, physical exam, complexity of medical decision-making, and/or time. These elements are broken down in Tables 5.1 to 5.5. The majority of initial observation

Table 5.1

Sample of E&M Documentation Options

Level	History	PE	MDM	Time	E&M
	Problem focused	Problem focused	Straightforward		99XXX
	Expanded problem focused	Expanded problem focused	Low		99XXX
	Detailed	Detailed	Moderate		99XXX
	Comprehensive	Comprehensive	High		99XXX

Table 5.2

History and Physical Exam Elaboration

History		Physical Exam	
Detailed	**Comprehensive**	**Detailed**	**Comprehensive**
– Chief complaint	– Chief complaint	At least 12 bullet points from any organ system	At least two bullet points from each of nine organ systems
– four HPI elements or the status of three chronic or inactive problems	– four HPI elements or the status of three chronic or inactive problems	**Organ Systems:** – Constitutional – Eyes – Ears/nose/ mouth/throat – Neck – Respiratory – Cardiovascular – Chest	– Abdomen – Genitourinary – Lymphatic – Musculoskeletal – Integumentary – Neurological – Psychiatric
– 2–9 systems in ROS	– 10 system ROS		
– ≥one element of PFSH	– Complete all three of PFSH		

HPI, history of present illness; PFSH, past family social history; ROS, review of systems.

and hospital care history and are either detailed or comprehensive and outlined in Tables 5.1 and 5.2. (Tables 5.6 through 5.10 provide additional details for the history and physical exam requirements.) Patients who are observation status or admitted routinely require comprehensive history and a physical exam. Get in the habit of always being thorough in your documentation and you will then consistently provide high-quality care that is billable at the highest levels.

Table 5.3

Medical Decision-Making Elaboration

Overall MDM	Presenting problem points	Complexity of data points	Risk of complication and/or morbidity/mortality
Straightforward	1	1	Minimal
Low complexity	2	2	Low
Moderate complexity	3	3	Moderate
High complexity	4	4	High

Table 5.4

Problem Points and Data Points Elaboration

Problem points		Data points	
Problem	Points	Data	Points
Self-limited or minor (max 2)	1	Review/order laboratory tests	1
Established problem/stable or improving (these may be multiplied by number of problems being treated	1	Review/order radiology test	1
Established problem, worsening (these may be multiplied by number of problems being treated	2	Review/order medical test	1
New problem, no additional workup planned (highest level is three no matter how many problems)	3	Discuss test with performing provider	1
New problem, additional workup planned (highest level is three no matter how many problems)	4	Independent review of image, tracing, or specimen	2
		Decision to obtain old records	1
		Review and summarize old records	2

Tables 5.3 and 5.4 and Exhibit 5.1 provide additional data to determine accurate medical decision-making levels. This takes time and practice but eventually will become second nature. Practice using these tables when in clinical, and discuss coding and billing with preceptors, as this is a critical skill to have in practice.

Table 5.5

Risk Elaboration (is determined by the risk related to the disease process anticipated between the present encounter and the next encounter)

Minimal	Lowest level of risk possible, not for inpatients Requires one element in any of the three categories: 1. Presenting problem • One self-limiting or minor problem 2. Diagnostic procedures/tests—examples: • CXR, EKG, EEG, UA • Ultrasound, ECHO 3. Management • Examples: rest, gargles, elastic bandages, superficial dressings
Low	Second lowest level of risk; Level I progress note, low-risk patients are generally quite healthy Requires one element in any of the three categories: 1. Presenting problem • One stable chronic illness • Acute, uncomplicated illness or injury 2. Diagnostic procedures/tests—examples: • Physiologic tests not under stress (e.g., pulmonary function tests (PFTs)) • Noncardiovascular imaging studies with contrast • Superficial needle biopsies • Arterial blood gas (ABGs) 3. Management • Over-the-counter medications • Minor surgery with no identified risk factors • Physical or occupational therapy • IV fluids without additives
Moderate	Second highest risk level—required for Level II hospital progress note Requires one element in any of the three categories: 1. Presenting problem • One or more chronic illnesses with mild exacerbation or progression • Two or more stable chronic illnesses • Undiagnosed problem with uncertain prognosis • Acute illness with systemic symptoms (e.g., pyelonephritis, pneumonitis, colitis) • Acute complicated injury (e.g., head injury with brief loss of consciousness) 2. Diagnostic procedures/tests—Examples: • Physiologic tests under stress (e.g., cardiac stress test) • Diagnostic endoscopies with no identified risk factors • Deep needle or incisional biopsies • Cardiovascular imaging studies with contrast and no identified risk factors (e.g., arteriogram, cardiac catheterization) • Obtain fluid from body cavity (e.g., lumbar puncture (LP), thoracentesis, paracentesis)

(continued)

Table 5.5

Risk Elaboration (is determined by the risk related to the disease process anticipated between the present encounter and the next encounter) (*continued*)

         3. Management—examples:
- Minor surgery with identified risk factors
- Elective major surgery with no risk factors
- Prescription drug management
- Therapeutic nuclear medicine
- IV fluids with additives
- Closed treatment of fracture or dislocation without manipulation

High   Highest level of risk, required for Level III admission

      Requires one element in any of the three categories:

      1. Presenting problem
- One or more chronic illnesses with severe exacerbation or progression
- Acute or chronic illness or injuries which pose a threat to life or bodily function (e.g., multiple trauma, acute MI, pulmonary embolism, severe respiratory distress, peritonitis, acute kidney injury)

      2. Diagnostic procedures/tests—examples:
- Cardiovascular imaging studies with contrast with identified risk factors
- Cardiac EP testing
- Diagnostic endoscopies with identified risk factors

      3. Management—examples
- Elective major surgery with identified risk factors
- Emergency major surgery
- Parenteral controlled substances
- Drug therapy requiring intensive monitoring for toxicity
- Decision not to resuscitate or to de-escalate care because of poor prognosis

PFT, pulmonary function test; ABG, arterial blood gas; LP, lumbar puncture.

Table 5.6

Documentation Elements for Billing Initial Hospital Care (requires all three of the History, Exam, and MDM to be met across the board or Time)

Level	History	PE	MDM	Time	E&M
1	Detailed	Detailed	Straightforward/low	30	99221
2	Comprehensive	Comprehensive	Moderate	50	99222
3	Comprehensive	Comprehensive	High	70	99223

E&M, evaluation and management code; MDM, medical decision-making; PE, physical exam; Time, displayed in minutes.

Table 5.7

Documentation Elements for Billing Initial Observation Care (requires all three of the History, Exam, and MDM to be met across the board or Time)

Level	History	PE	MDM	Time	E&M
1	Detailed	Detailed	Straightforward/low	30	99218
2	Comprehensive	Comprehensive	Moderate	50	99219
3	Comprehensive	Comprehensive	High	70	99220

E&M, evaluation and management code; MDM, medical decision-making; PE, physical exam; Time, displayed in minutes.

Table 5.8

Documentation Elements for Billing Initial Observation With Discharge on Same Date of Service (requires all three of the History, Exam, and MDM to be met across the board or Time)

Level	History	PE	MDM	Time	E&M
1	Detailed	Detailed	Straightforward/low	40	99234
2	Comprehensive	Comprehensive	Moderate	50	99235
3	Comprehensive	Comprehensive	High	55	99236

E&M, evaluation and management code; MDM, medical decision-making; PE, physical exam; Time, displayed in minutes.

Table 5.9

Documentation Elements for Billing Subsequent Care (requires two of the three of the History, Exam, and MDM to be met or Time, or can be based on time if time spent bedside >50% spent coordinating care)

Level	Patient	History	PE	MDM	Time	E&M
1	Stable or improving	Problem focused	Problem focused	Straightforward/low	15	99231
2	Inadequate response to treatment or minor complication	Expanded problem focused	Expanded problem focused	Moderate	25	99232

(continued)

Table 5.9

Documentation Elements for Billing Subsequent Care (requires two of the three of the History, Exam, and MDM to be met or Time, or can be based on time if time spent bedside >50% spent coordinating care) (*continued*)

Level	Patient	History	PE	MDM	Time	E&M
3	Unstable or has significant complication or a significant new problem	Detailed	Detailed	High	35	99233

E&M, evaluation and management code; MDM, medical decision-making; PE, physical exam; Time, displayed in minutes.

Table 5.10

Documentation Elements for Billing Subsequent Observation (care requires two of the three of the History, Exam, and MDM to be met or Time)

Level	Patient	History	PE	MDM	Time	E&M
1	Stable or improving	Problem focused	Problem focused	Straightforward/low	15	99224
2	Inadequate response to treatment or minor complication	Expanded problem focused	Expanded problem focused	Moderate	25	99225
3	Unstable or has significant complication or a significant new problem	Detailed	Detailed	High	35	99226

E&M, evaluation and management code; MDM, medical decision-making; PE, physical exam; Time, displayed in minutes.

Table 5.11

	Documentation Elements for Consultation Billing (requires all three of the History, Exam, and MDM to be met across the board or Time)				
Level	History	PE	MDM	Time	E&M
1	Problem focused	Problem focused	Straightforward	20	99251
2	Expanded problem focused	Expanded problem focused	Straightforward	40	99252
3	Detailed	Detailed	Low	55	99253
4	Comprehensive	Comprehensive	Moderate	80	99254
5	Comprehensive	Comprehensive	High	110	99255

E&M, evaluation and management code; MDM, medical decision-making; PE, physical exam; Time, displayed in minutes.

Medical Decision-Making (MDM)

Three elements are required to determine medical decision-making. Problem points, data points, and risk assessment comprise the overall MDM. The MDM score is two out of three/average of the three areas in Table 5.3. Example: A patient scores low or 2 points for complexity of data points and high complexity for presenting problem points; the average is moderate complexity for the overall MDM. Most hospitalized patients are moderate- or high-complexity MDM. Each of the problem points and data points are elaborated upon in Table 5.4, and risk stratification is elaborated upon in Table 5.5.

Consultations

NPs can work on teams that provide consultative services, such as infectious disease, cardiology, nephrology, palliative care, and so forth. These consultations require different codes since the consulting provider is not the admitting team in this situation (see Table 5.11). NPs may not bill for a consult that determines the need for surgery if that surgery/procedures falls outside their scope of practice.

Fast Facts

Get in the habit of always being thorough in your documentation and you will then consistently provide high-quality care that is billable at the higher levels.

Critical Care Billing

Critical care codes are time-based billing and used for any life-, limb-, or organ-saving interventions. Record the total time spent evaluating, managing, providing care, and documenting such activities. This includes time taken to

- complete chart review,
- perform a history and physical exam,
- interpret laboratory and diagnostic testing,
- consider differential diagnoses,
- develop a working diagnosis,
- develop and implement a plan of care, and
- document.

Time spent can be at the bedside, discussing the case with staff, documenting the medical record, and time spent with family members (or MDM) discussing specific treatment issues and decisions. During this time the NP must devote his or her full attention to this particular patient.

Critical care time is not solely billable for ICU patients or by ICU providers. Critical care time can be billed by any AG-ACNP for any urgent or emergent situation to assess, manipulate, and support vital organ systems and/or to prevent further life-threatening deterioration of the patient's condition. Examples include rapid-response activations for hemodynamic instability; unstable cardiac rhythm such as rapid atrial fibrillation; hypoxic or hypercarbic respiratory failure; code stroke; ST elevated myocardial infarction (STEMI) alert; sepsis alerts; and so forth where high-complexity medical decision-making is utilized to diagnose and stabilization is performed. CMS adds that to qualify as critical care, the failure to initiate these interventions on an urgent basis would likely result in sudden, clinically significant or life-threatening deterioration.

Fast Facts

Critical care is time-based billing for any life-, limb-, or organ-saving interventions.

The two critical care codes are 99291 for the first hour, but may be billed after the halfway threshold has been met at 30 minutes, and 99292 for each additional 30 minutes beyond the initial hour, but may be billed once the halfway threshold has been met at 75 minutes. Functions are NOT to be included in this are

- time for procedures,
- routine daily family updates, and
- professional services for interpretation of diagnostic testing.

While NPs routinely interpret EKGs and CXRs, the cardiologist and radiologists are the qualified experts who bill for the professional services to provide the "final read" on these diagnostic tests. Daily family updates are expected elements of the care provided; however, formal family meetings, where care decisions are made, can be billed as critical care time. Decisions such as making the patient "do not resuscitate" (DNR) or withdrawing interventions to focus on comfort care are important to clearly document and are considered billable time. Of note, the family's decision to continue current therapies is also a conscious decision and should be recorded as such.

Fast Facts

Please note that Medicare rules can vary or change from region to region based on the local Medicare carrier. Be sure to check with your billing staff, who know more specifics.

Prolonged Services

Prolonged services are designed for times when coordinating care is time-consuming. To bill the E&M code 99356 requires additional >60-minute increments of face-to-face time with the patient for the NP beyond the initial or subsequent care codes for the day (this first unit may be billed after the halfway mark threshold has been met, minimum of 30 minutes in prolonged care time may be billed). Additional increments of >30-minute increments (beyond the first hour) can be billed using code 99357.

For successful reimbursement, the NP must record the time in and out of the patient room ,including start and stop time, and list the care and coordination or discussion that occurred during each entrance to the patient's room. The following CANNOT be billed as prolonged services:

- time spent reviewing the patient chart
- discussing the patient with residents or nursing staff that is not direct face-to-face contact with the patient
- awaiting diagnostic results
- managing changes in the patient's condition

Of note, Medicare states: "While Medicare recognizes the effort that goes into prolonged services, it doesn't expect to see the codes used very often."

Discharges

- Patients who are admitted and discharged on the same calendar date as observation status would use codes 99234, 99235, and 99236 as listed in Table 5.8.

- For patients who are discharged from observation on a different day than they were admitted for observation, the NP should use code 99217.
- Inpatient discharge:
  - Less than 30 minutes, use code 99238.
  - Greater than 30 minutes, use code 99239.
  - Note that specific time must be documented as well as the discharge day services that were performed.
  - Discharges codes may be used in the event of death pronouncement.

Coding and Billing Tips

- Get to know the coding specialist for the department. Take time to meet them and ask questions. They are there to educate and support you. They are more than happy to answer your questions.
- Anticipate a review of your documentation and coaching to meet the documentation requirements.
- Respond quickly and accurately to the coder's clinical queries or requests for additional documentation or clarification.
- Discuss billing with the attending of record on a daily basis.
- Attend all annual or semiannual training requirements. Come with questions and examples to discuss.

Fast Facts

Changes to inpatient coding and billing are anticipated for 2023. Be sure to attend the required coding and billing training per your institutional policy.

Reimbursement

Reimbursement is a separate concept from billing. Reimbursement is quite complex and beyond the scope of this book and out of the control of NPs. Simply put, documentation must support the billing submitted. Additionally, billing for a service does not necessarily mean it will be reimbursed. The group practice is reimbursed for NP services by CMS and other insurance companies and is typically reimbursed at 85% of physician rates.

In summary, learning to code and bill for services can be daunting; however, with practice and determination, you can provide quality patient care while augmenting the institutional finances. Be sure to build a relationship with your department billing and coding specialists. Respond promptly to requests for clarification and additional documentation.

References

The Change Over from ICD-9-CM to ICD-10-CM. (2021). *MedicalCodingand Billing.org*. www.medicalbillingandcoding.org/icd-10-cm/

CMS. (2020, 23 December 2020). *MS-DRG Classifications and Software*. www.cms .gov/Medicare/Medicare-Fee-for-Service-Payment/AcuteInpatientPPS/ MS-DRG-Classifications-and-Software

MM5972 Prolonged Services (Codes 99354–99359). (2017, 7 March 2017). www .cms.gov/Outreach-and-Education/Medicare-Learning-Network-MLN/ MLNMattersArticles/downloads/mm5972.pdf

Dean, S. M., Gilmore-Bykovskyi, A., Buchanan, J., Ehlenfeldt, B., & Kind, A. J. (2016). Design and hospital-wide implementation of a standardized discharge summary in an electronic health record. *The Joint Commission Journal on Quality and Patient Safety*, *42*(12), 555–AP11.

Sanderson, A. L., & Burns, J. P. (2020). Clinical documentation for intensivists: The impact of diagnosis documentation. *Critical Care Medicine*, *48*(4), 579–587.

CMS. (2018). *Are you a hospital inpatient or outpatient? CMS*. www.medicare .gov/Pubs/pdf/11435-Are-You-an-Inpatient-or-Outpatient.pdf

6

Fluids, Electrolytes, Nutrition

Prescribing intravenous fluids, electrolytes, and nutrition is routine for acute care nurse practitioners. Understanding the risks, benefits, and alternatives is essential to providing quality care. While prescribing electrolytes can become a routine intervention, being cognizant of conditions that require limits or changes to these interventions is key to prevent worsening a clinical scenario.

In this chapter, you will learn

- the differences between types of intravenous fluids,
- how to replenish electrolytes,
- how to calculate caloric needs and tube-feeding rates,
- how to calculate parenteral nutrition, and
- how to recognize refeeding syndrome.

INTRAVENOUS (IV) FLUIDS

Almost all inpatients receive IV fluids of some sort at some point during their stay. IV fluids play a distinct role in attaining and maintaining euvolemia. They do, however, have side effects and can cause harm if they are not fully understood. First and foremost is understanding the osmolality and electrolyte components of each fluid. Tables 6.1 and 6.2 review the osmolality and electrolyte components of commonly prescribed crystalloid and colloid IV fluids.

Table 6.1

Crystalloid Fluid Comparison Chart

Solution	Osmo	pH	Na+	Cl−	K+	Ca+	Glucose	Other
NS**	308	6.0	154	154	−	−	−	
¼ NS*	86	6.0	39	39	−	−	−	
½ NS*	154	6.0	77	77	−	−	−	
3% NS***	1,026	5.0	513	513	−	−	−	
LR**	273	6.5	130	109	4	3	−	Lactate 28 mEq/L
Plasmalyte**	294	7.4	140	98	5	3	−	Acetate 27 mEq/L Gluconate 23 mEq/L
D5W*	253	4.5	−	−	−	−	50	=170 kcal/L
D10%W***	505	4.3	−	−	−	−	100	=340 kcal/L
D5W ½ NS***	432	4.0	77	77	−	−	50	=170 kcal/L
D5NS***	560	4.4	154	154	−	−	50	=170 kcal/L
D5WLR***	525	5.0	130	109	4	3	50	
7.5% NaHCO3***	1,786	8.0	893	−	−	−	−	HCO3 893

*Hypotonic, **Isotonic, ***Hypertonic.
Osmo = Osmolarity in mOsm/L; Electrolytes in mEq/L; Glucose in g/L.

Table 6.2

Colloid Fluid Comparison Chart							
Solution	Osmo	pH	Na$^+$	Cl$^-$	K$^+$	Ca$^+$	Glucose	Other
Albumin 5%	330	7.4	145	–	≤2	–	–	Albumin 50 g/L
Albumin 25%	330	7.4	145	–	≤2	–	–	Albumin 250 g/L
10% Dextran 40 in NS	308	4.0	154	154	–	–	–	Dextran 100 g/L
Hetastarch 6% in NS	308	5.9	154	154	–	–	–	Hetastarch 60 g/L

Fast Facts

Hypotonic fluids should never be given to any patient who has or is suspected of having cerebral edema, acute traumatic brain injury, seizures, or stroke.

ELECTROLYTES

Calculate Corrected Levels of Electrolytes

Corrected Serum Calcium level

Is used in patients with hypoalbuminemia.
Corrected calcium (mg/dL) = measured total Ca (mg/dL) + .8 (4.0 – serum albumin [g/dL]), where 4.0 represents the average albumin level.

Corrected Serum Sodium level

Is used in patients with severe hyperglycemia as in diabetic ketoacidosis (DKA) or hyperglycemic hyperosmolar syndrome (HHS).
Corrected sodium = measured sodium + (1.6 [glucose – 100]/100).

Repletion of Electrolytes

The following are guidelines for replacement of electrolytes (see Tables 6.3–6.6). Customize to patient needs. These guidelines apply to adult patients:

- >40 kilograms and
- whose creatinine clearance is >30 mL/min,
- with a serum creatinine <2.0, and
- urine output >30 mL/hr

Table 6.3

Hypokalemia Replacement

Serum potassium (mmol/L)	Potassium chloride Oral route preferred if able IV doses are for central line
3.8–3.9	KCL 20 mEq PO or IVPB × 1
3.5–3.7	KCL 20 mEq PO Q 2 hours × 2 doses or 20 mEq IVPB Q 1 hour × 2
3.0–3.4	KCL 40 mEq PO, then 2 hours later give 20 mEq PO to total 60 mEq or KCL 20 mEq over 1 hour × 3 for a total of 60 mEq
<3.0	KCL 20 mEq over 1 hour × 4 for a total of 80 mEq
Repeat serum potassium level 2 hours after last doses completed.	

IVPB, intravenous piggyback.

Table 6.4

Hypomagnesemia Replacement

Serum magnesium (mg/dL)	Magnesium sulfate
1.7–2.0	2 g IVPB over 1 hour
1.2–1.6	4 g IVPB over 2 hours
<1.2	6 g IVPB over 3 hours
Repeat serum magnesium level 2 hours after last doses completed.	

Table 6.5

Hypophosphatemia Replacement

Serum phosphate (Mg/dL)	Sodium or potassium phosphate
2.0–2.4	Neutra-Phos one packet PO Q 6 hours for 48 hours Sodium or potassium phosphate 15 mmol IV over 6 hours
1.5–1.9	Neutra-Phos two packets PO Q 6 hours for 48 hours or Sodium or potassium phosphate 30 mmol IV over 6 hours
<1.5	Sodium or potassium phosphate 45 mmol IV over 6 hours
Repeat serum phosphorus level 2 hours after last doses completed.	

Note: Potassium phosphate is used when the patient is also hypokalemic.

Table 6.6

Hypocalcemia	
Ionized serum calcium (mmol/L)	Calcium gluconate
1–1.12	2 g IVPB over 2 hours
<1.0	4 g IVPB over 4 hours
Repeat serum ionized calcium level 2 hours after last doses completed.	

Note: Consider dose adjustments in patients with hyperphosphatemia, severe acidosis, patients receiving digoxin, or on continuous renal replacement therapy.

Fast Facts

Remember, it's easier to give additional supplementation than to get it back if too much is given. Smaller doses given more frequently is better than being too aggressive initially.

Fast Facts

Use extreme caution when prescribing potassium, phosphorus, and magnesium in patients with acute kidney injury or end-stage renal disease.

Hyponatremia

Acute hyponatremia is defined as documented as lasting less than 48 hours, whereas chronic hyponatremia is defined as documented lasting greater than 48 hours. Mild hyponatremia is classified as 130 to 135 mmol/L; moderate, 125 to 129 mmol/L; and profound, <125 mmol/L. Hyperglycemic hypernatremia should be corrected using corrected serum sodium levels. Corrected serum sodium = measured Na + 2.4 × ([glucose − 100 mg/dL]/100 mg/dL).

Sodium correction:

Slowly correct by .5 mmol/L per hour and not more than 6 mmol/L per 24 hours.

.9% NS = 154 mmol sodium chloride.

3% NS = 513% Sodium chloride.

Correcting hyponatremia too quickly can lead to osmotic demyelination syndrome (ODS), which can lead to permanent brain damage. Central pontine myelinolysis (CPM) most commonly damages the pons, whereas extrapontine myelinolysis (EPM) damages other parts of the brain. About 10% of those with CPM will have EPM. Symptoms begin to appear 2 to 3 days after correction of the sodium level and include dysarthria, dysphagia, muscle weakness of the limbs, confusion, decreased level of consciousness, and seizures. The most severe cases of central pontine myelinolysis can result in locked-in syndrome.

NUTRITION

Critically ill patients who are malnourished are associated with poor outcomes, including higher mortality rates, impaired wound healing, and greater rate of nosocomial infections. Assessment of nutritional status should be done within the first 24 hours of admission. The first nutritional risk assessment tool developed and validated specifically for ICU patients is the NUTRIC score. To calculate the NUTRIC score, use Table 6.7, and to interpret the results, use Table 6.8.

Critically ill patients should receive nutrition within the first 24 hours of admission. Ideally, enteral feeding via the GI tract is the safest and most economical. Waiting for the nutritionist to write recommendations is not efficient; thus, NPs need to be able to start tube-feeding on

Table 6.7

NUTRIC Score		
Variable	Range	Points
Age	<50	0
	50–<75	1
	≥75	2
APACHE II score	<15	0
	15–<20	1
	20–28	2
	>28	3
SOFA score	<6	0
	6–<10	1
	≥10	2
Number of comorbidities	0–1	0
	≥2	1
Days from hospital to ICU admission	0–≤1	0
	≥1	1
IL-6	0–<400	0
	≥400	1

Table 6.8

NUTRIC Score Interpretation

Interpretation of NUTRIC score with IL-6:

Sum of points	Category	Explanation
6–10	High score	Associated with worse clinical outcomes (e.g., mortality, ventilation). Most likely to benefit from aggressive nutrition therapy.
0–5	Low score	These patients have low malnutrition risk.

NUTRIC score without IL-6:

Sum of points	Category	Explanation
5–9	High score	Associated with worse clinical outcomes (e.g., mortality, ventilation). Most likely to benefit from aggressive nutrition therapy.
0–4	Low score	These patients have low malnutrition risk.

their own. Critically ill patients typically require 25 or more kilocalories (kcal) per kilogram per day. Protein requirements typically average 1.2 to 2 grams per kilogram per day.

For both tube-feeding and parenteral nutritional calculations, the first step is to calculate the feeding weight (FW). Feeding patients at their ideal body weight would underfeed an overweight patient. And conversely, feeding the patient's actual body weight (ABW) would be too many calories and lead to overfeeding and other complications. Thus, we need to allow for additional nutrition to feed the extra muscle mass that is required to carry the extra weight when patients are overweight.

The following are merely rough estimates to facilitate early nutrition within the first 24 hours. Consult nutritionist for more specific targets based on individual patient needs.

Calculate Caloric Goals

- Calculate Ideal Body Weight (IBW) =
  - For women, start with 48 kg and add 2.2 kg for each inch over 5′ tall
  - For men, start with 50 kg and add 2.2 kg for each inch over 5′ tall
  - Example: woman at $5'6'' = 48 + (6 \times 2.2) = 61.2$ kg IBW
- Calculate Feeding Weight (FW) = (ABW – IBW)/4 + IBW
  - Example: Woman at 61.2 kg IBW whose ABW is 80 kg
  - $(80 \text{ kg} - 61.2 \text{ kg})/4 + 61.2 = 65.9$ kg FW
- Daily Caloric Goal = Feeding weight × 25 kcal
  - Example: FW of 65.9 kg × 25 kcal = 1,647.5 calories/day

Tube-Feeding (TF) Calculations

- Goal TF = caloric goal/24 hours.
- Example: 1,648 calories per day/24 hours = 68.67 calories/hour.
- Thus, if TF is one cal/mL, then the TF rate would be 68 mL/hr; OK to round to 70 mL/hr.
- Adjust rate based on concentration of calories per mL of TF.
- Example: If TF is 2 cal/mL, then the infusion rate would be 35 mL/hr.
- Example: If TF is 1.5 cal/mL, then the infusion rate would be ~52 or 53 mL/hr.

Fast Facts

Enteral feedings should be used if the patient has a functioning gastrointestinal tract.

Parenteral Nutrition

The following are merely rough estimates to facilitate parenteral nutrition when a nutritionist may not be readily available to provide specific recommendations based on individual patient needs:

1. Calculate caloric needs per day based on feeding weight.
2. Calculate protein needs:
   a. .8–1 g/kg for renal failure patients not yet on HD
   b. 1.2 g/kg for renal failure patients now on HD
   c. 1.5 g/kg for all other patients
   d. Calculate protein calories = # grams total × 4 kcal/g
3. Calculate lipid needs:
   a. Be sure to document triglyceride level <350 before adding lipids.
   b. (Total calories – protein calories) × 1/3 = total lipid calories.
   c. 1 g lipid – 9 kcal.
   d. Total lipid calories/9 = gram lipid needed.
4. Carbohydrate (CHO) needs (dextrose):
   a. Total caloric need – (protein calories + lipid calories) = CHO calories.
   b. CHO calories/3.4 kcal = CHO grams needed.
   c. Be SURE that CHO total does NOT exceed 2–4 g CHO/kg/min.
   d. Start with maximum 200 g dextrose in first 24 hours and increase by ~50 g/d until goal is reached.
   e. Consequence of too much dextrose is hyperglycemia and the need for additional insulin, thus causing hypokalemia from the extra dextrose and insulin.

Fast Facts

To be able to calculate parenteral nutrition (PN), the nurse practitioner needs to know how many kilocalories are in each gram of the three nutritional components of PN.

- Protein: 4 kilocalories per gram of protein
- Fat: 9 kilocalories per gram of fat
- Carbohydrates: 3.4 kilocalories per gram of carbohydrate

5. Monitoring:
   a. Check chemistries daily until stable.
   b. Frequent finger stick blood glucose until stable on PN.
   c. With long-term PN, watch for signs of sepsis, including fungemia.
6. Additives:
   a. Can add multivitamins, thiamine, folate (as available based on national shortages).
   b. Electrolytes: Do not use PN to replenish low electrolyte levels, as patient will need to wait for a new bag to be hung, which is usually later in the day. Providers can add slowly as ongoing needs and daily repletion are noted over a few days to a week.
   c. Can add heparin for DVT prophylaxis and H2 blockers such as Pepcid for stress ulcer prophylaxis; however, check with your institutional policies
   d. Can add insulin to PN; however, exercise caution in the acute phase, as it may cause hypoglycemia, and then the only way to remedy this is to waste the bag of PN. It is recommended to keep insulin separate from PN until stable doses of PN and insulin are established after a week in a stable state.

Fast Facts

Do not use PN to replete electrolyte levels, as this is not timely; the patient will need to wait for a new bag to be hung, which can be hours later.

Refeeding Syndrome

Patients who are underweight or severely malnourished are at risk for refeeding syndrome. The hallmark sign of refeeding syndrome is hypophosphatemia that occurs within 12 to 24 hours of initiation of nutrition.

Severe hypophosphatemia <1.0 can cause respiratory insufficiency and respiratory arrest. Thus, aggressive repletion of phosphorus is required in addition to slow progression of feedings over days to weeks to get to the goal.

Fast Facts

The hallmark sign of refeeding syndrome is hypophosphatemia. Severe hypophosphatemia can cause respiratory depression. Refeeding syndrome requires aggressive IV repletion.

In summary, prescribing and managing fluids, electrolytes, and nutrition are foundational knowledge and skills for the AG-ACNP to possess. It takes practice to master the skill. Consult with colleagues, pharmacists, and nutritionists to ensure patient needs are adequately met without exceeding patient needs.

References

de Vries, M. C., Koekkoek, W. K., Opdam, M. H., van Blokland, D., & van Zanten, A. R. (2018). Nutritional assessment of critically ill patients: validation of the modified NUTRIC score. *European Journal of Clinical Nutrition*, *72*(3), 428–435.

George, J. C., Zafer, W., Bucaloiu, I. D., & Chang, A. R. (2018). Risk factors and outcomes of rapid correction of severe hyponatremia. *Clinical Journal of the American Society of Nephrology*, *13*(7), 984–992. https://doi.org/10.2215/CJN.13061117

Nexus, M. *Quarter normal saline*. www.mdnxs.com/topics-2/pharmacology/quarter-normal-saline/

Louisiana State University Health Care Services Division. (2009). *Adult electrolyte replacement protocol*. www.medschool.lsuhsc.edu/emergency_medicine/docs/adult%20electrolyte%20replacement%20protocol%20-%20mcln%200006%20j.pdf

NIH. (27 March 2019). *Central pontine myelinolysis information page*. National Institute of Neurological Disorders and Stroke. www.ninds.nih.gov/disorders/all-disorders/central-pontine-myelinolysis-information-page

II

Body Systems

7

Neurological Acute Care

The neurological system can often be challenging to learn and recall. The most important elements the AG-ACNP needs to master are anatomy and a thorough neurological exam. Recognition of neurological deficits early is critical to activating emergency neurological life-support teams, thus saving brain tissue, maintaining function, and preserving independent living.

In this chapter, you will learn

- anatomy of the cerebral vasculature,
- cranial nerve anatomy and function,
- dermatome levels,
- to differentiate between types of pain,
- National Institute of Health (NIH) stroke assessment and care,
- contraindications and relative contraindications to tissue plasminogen activator (TPA), and
- brain-death criteria.

ANATOMY

Understanding the anatomy, physiology, and function of the brain and spinal cord is essential to understanding the signs and symptoms of disease processes and injury patterns. The circle of Willis defines the vasculature and is important to understand patterns of deficits seen with ischemic strokes (see Figure 7.1). Cranial nerves and dermatomes are important to assess for neurological deficits (see Table 7.1 and Figures 7.2 and 7.3). Unless an AG-ACNP elects to work with a neurology, neurosurgical, or neuro-critical care team, recalling these items requires frequent review to master.

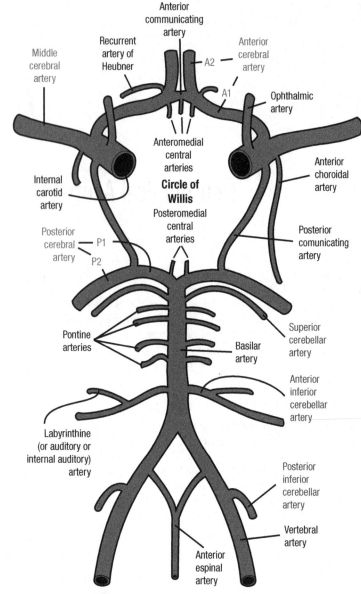

Figure 7.1 Circle of Willis

Source: Courtesy of R. H. Castilhos.

Table 7.1

Cranial nerves	Name	Mnemonic	Function	Motor or sensory	Mnemonic
I	Olfactory	On	Smell	Sensory	Some
II	Optic	Old	Sight	Sensory	Say
III	Oculomotor	Olympus	Eye movement	Motor	Marry
IV	Trochlear	Towering	Eye movement	Motor	Money
V	Trigeminal	Tops	Facial sensation and movement	Both	But
VI	Abducens	A	Eye movement	Motor	My
VII	Facial	Fin	Face: expression and sensory	Both	Brother
VIII	Acoustic (Vestibulocochlear)	And	Hearing & balance	Sensory	Says
IX	Glossopharyngeal	German	Tongue and Throat	Both	Bad
X	Vagus	Viewed	Parasympathetic	Both	Business
XI	Spinal Accessory	Some	Head, neck; shoulder movement and swallow	Motor	Marries
XII	Hypoglossal	Hops	Speech, chewing and swallowing	Motor	Money

DERMATOMES

Subarachnoid Hemorrhages

Classic signs of an aneurysmal subarachnoid hemorrhage (SAH) include a report of a severe headache with a rapid/abrupt onset, often referred to as a "thunderclap" headache. The headache is commonly described as pulsatile, and some patients report hearing blood rushing. Associated symptoms include the following:

- vomiting
- decreased level of consciousness
- hemiparesis
- seizures
- neck stiffness that occurs about 6 hours after headache onset

Exam findings of meningeal irritation include Kernig sign (inability to fully extend the knees when the thigh is flexed at the hip and knee is at a 90-degree angle) and Brudzinski sign (hip and knee flexion with

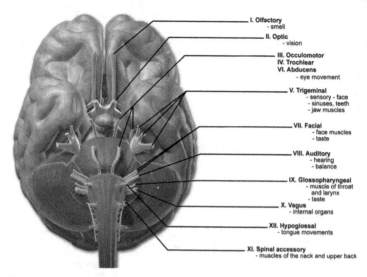

Figure 7.2   Cranial nerves

Source: Courtesy of Bruce Blausen.

passive neck flexion). Management of SAH is focused on monitoring for and prevention of rebleeding and vasospasm (see Tables 7.2 and 7.3).

Predicting Outcomes of Intracranial Hemorrhage

A frequent question by families of patients with intracranial hemorrhage is "What will be their outcome?" Two scoring systems can be used to aid clinicians in predicting outcomes. The Intracranial Hemorrhage score (ICH) grades the ICH severity and predicts mortality at 30 days. Whereas, the Functional Outcome in Patients with Primary Intracerebral Hemorrhage (FUNC) score identifies patients with intracranial hemorrhage who are likely to attain functional independence at 90 days postadmission. These scores can be used to help guide goals of care discussions with patients and their families (see Table 7.4).

Treatment of Intracranial Bleeding

The cornerstone of treatment for all intracranial bleeding includes the reversal of coagulopathies and blood pressure (BP) control. Patients with ICH should have a neurosurgical consult. Blood pressure goals can vary by neurosurgeon and neurocritical care providers. Cardene and labetalol drips are commonly used to achieve blood pressure goals quickly and avoid swings in blood pressure. Ensure blood pressure goals are well documented in both the order set and progress notes. See Hematology chapter (Chapter 12) for anticoagulation reversal agents and dosing.

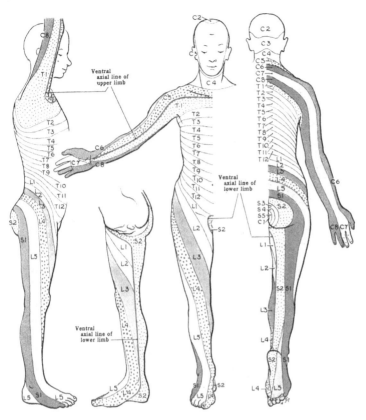

Figure 7.3   Dermatome man

Source: Courtesy of John Charles Boileau Grant., https://commons.wikimedia.
org/wiki/File:Grant_1962_663.png

Table 7.2

Hunt and Hess Grading Scale for SAH—Used to Predict Outcome		
Grade	Criteria	Exam
1	Asymptomatic or mild headache	Minimal nuchal rigidity
2	Moderate to severe headache	Nuchal rigidity
3	Drowsiness or confusion	Mild focal neurological deficits
4	Stupor	Moderate to severe hemiparesis
5	Coma	Decerebrate posturing

SAH, subarachnoid hemorrhage.

Table 7.3

Modified Fisher Grading Scale for SAH—Used to Predict Risk of Cerebral Arterial Vasospasm

Grade	Criteria
0	No SAH or IVH
1	Minimal SAH; no IVH in the lateral two ventricles
2	Minimal SAH; IVH in the lateral two ventricles
3	Large SAH completely filling one or more cisterna or fissure; no IVH in the two lateral ventricles
4	Large SAH completely filling one or more cisterna or fissure; IVH in the two lateral ventricles

IVH, intraventricular hemorrhage; SAH, subarachnoid hemorrhage.

Table 7.4

Comparison of Tools to Predict Outcomes of ICH

ICH		FUNC	
Predicts ICH associated mortality at 30 days		**Predicts functional independence at 90 days**	
Criteria	Points	Criteria	Points
ICH volume in cm3		ICH volume in cm3	
– >30	1	– <30	4
– <30	0	– 30–60	2
		– >60	0
Age		Age	
– >80	1	– <70	2
– <80	0	– 70–79	1
		– ≥80	0
Location		Location	
– Infratentorial	1	– Lobar	2
– Supratentorial	0	– Deep	1
		– Infratentorial	0
GCS		GCS score	
– 3–4	2	– ≥9	1
– 5–12	1	– ≤8	0
– 13–15	0		
Intraventricular blood		Pre-ICH cognitive impairment	
– Yes	1	– No	1
– No	0	– Yes	0

(continued)

Table 7.4

Comparison of Tools to Predict Outcomes of ICH (*continued*)	
ICH	**FUNC**
Predicts ICH associated mortality at 30 days	**Predicts functional independence at 90 days**
Interpretation: percent of mortality at 30 days: – Score 0 = 0% – Score 1 = 13% – Score 2 = 26% – Score 3 = 72% – Score 4 = 97% – Score 5 or 6 = 100%	Interpretation: percent who achieve functional independence by 90 days: – 0–4 = 0% – 5–7 = 1–20% – 8 = 21–60% – 9–10 = 61–80% – 11 = 81–100%

FUNC, functional outcome in patients with primary intracerebral hemorrhage; GCS, Glasgow Coma Scale; ICH, intracranial hemorrhage score.

CORRECTED PHENYTOIN (DILANTIN) LEVEL

Many patients with traumatic or aneurysmal SAH are at higher risk for seizures. Phenytoin has a narrow therapeutic index, thus monitoring is indicated. Phenytoin readily binds to albumin, and only the free phenytoin is able to cross the blood-brain barrier. Free phenytoin (Dilantin) level is preferred when available, however is costlier. Thus, for patients with hypoalbuminemia, calculating the corrected phenytoin level must be used to account for the reduced phenytoin protein.

Corrected phenytoin level = (Measured phenytoin) .25* Albumin + .1

ISCHEMIC STROKE

An ischemic stroke is the most common type of stroke.

Fast Facts

The mnemonic for ischemic stroke is "BE FAST": Balance (loss of balance, dizziness, headache), Eyes (blurry vision), Face (facial droop), Arms (Arm or leg weakness), Speech (dysarthria), Time (call 911 or a code stroke/brain attack if in hospital).

A "Code Stroke" or "Brain Attack" should be called over the hospital emergency system as soon as signs/symptoms are recognized in inpatients. A CT scan of the brain should be completed within 25 minutes of arrival or symptom onset and interpreted within 45 minutes. National Institutes of Health Stroke Scale (NIHSS) should be performed immediately (see Table 7.5).

Table 7.5

National Institutes of Health Stroke Scale		
1a.	LOC	0 – alert; keenly responsive 1 – not alert, but arousable with minor stimulation 2 – not alert; requires repeated stimulation 3 – unresponsive or only with reflexes
1b.	LOC questions: – What is the month? - What is your age?	0 – answers both questions correctly 1 – answers one question correctly 3 – answers neither question correctly
1c.	LOC commands: - Open/close your eyes. - Grip/release your hand.	0 – Performs both tasks correctly 1 – Performs one task correctly 2 – Performs neither task correctly
2.	Best gaze	0 – Normal 1 – Partial gaze palsy 2 – Forced deviation
3.	Visual	0 – No visual loss 1 – Partial hemianopia 2 – Complete hemianopia 3 – Bilateral hemianopia
4.	Facial palsy	0 – Normal symmetric movements 1 – Minor paralysis 2 – Partial paralysis 3 – Complete paralysis of one or both sides
5.	Motor arms: a. Left b. Right	0 – No drift 1 – Drift 2 – Some effort against gravity 3 – No effort against gravity; limb falls 4 – No movement
6.	Motor legs: a. Left b. Right	0 – No drift 1 – Drift 2 – Some effort against gravity 3 – No effort against gravity; limb falls 4 – No movement

(continued)

Table 7.5

National Institutes of Health Stroke Scale (*continued*)		
7.	Limb Ataxia	0 – Absent 1 – Present in one limb 2 – Present in both limbs
8.	Sensory	0 – Normal 1 – Mild to moderate sensory loss 2 – Severe to total sensory loss
9.	Best Language	0 – Normal 1 – Mild to moderate aphasia 2 – Severe aphasia 3 – global aphasia
10.	Dysarthria	0 – Normal speech 1 – Mild to moderate dysarthria 2 – Severe dysarthria
11.	Extinction and inattention	0 – No abnormality 1 – Visual/tactile/auditory/spatial or personal inattention 2 – Profound hemi-inattention or extinction

LOC, level of consciousness.

Thrombolytics

- First ensure patient is not hypoglycemic or hypothermic, as hypoglycemia can mimic these stroke symptoms.
- Blood pressure goals before administration: SBP <185 and DBP <110.
- Consider use of labetalol 10–20 mg IV boluses, or nicardipine or clevidipine infusions.

  rtPA (alteplase)

- .9 mg/kg, maximum dose 90 mg with initial 10% of dose given as bolus over 1 minute and the remainder over 60 minutes
- Given within 3 hours of onset of stroke symptoms or the last time the patient was known to be well
- rtPA can be given up to 4.5 hours but commonly excludes:
  - patients over age 80,
  - patients taking warfarin,
  - patients with history of diabetes mellitus and previous ischemic stroke, and
  - patients with NIHSS score >25 because of an increased risk of intracranial bleeding.
- Consider mechanical thrombectomy if symptoms do not resolve quickly.

Tenecteplase administration is an alternative to rtPA (single IV bolus of .25 mg/kg, maximum 25 mg) in patients without contraindications for IV fibrinolysis who are also eligible to undergo mechanical thrombectomy (see Table 7.6).

Endovascular Therapy

After thrombolytics are given, noninvasive intracranial vascular imaging should be immediately obtained. Patients should receive mechanical thrombectomy with a stent retriever if they meet criteria. Maximal benefit is seen when reperfusion to TICI grade 2b/three is obtained within 6 hours of stroke onset (see Table 7.7).

Post-Thrombolytic Administration

- BP goal SBP <180/105.
- Hold ASA and DVT prophylaxis for 24 hours after thrombolytic administration.

Table 7.6

Contraindications and Relative Contraindications for rTPA	
Contraindications	**Relative contraindications**
• NIHSS 0-5	• Wake up after unknown downtime
• CT with intracranial hemorrhage	• Dural puncture within 7 days
• Ischemic stroke within 3 months	• Arterial puncture within 7 days
• Severe head trauma within 3 months	• Major surgery within 14 days
• Intracranial/intraspinal surgery within 3 months	• Major trauma not involving head trauma within 14 days
• Subarachnoid hemorrhage	• Intracranial arterial dissection
• GI malignancy or GI bleed within 21 days	• Unruptured intracranial aneurysms
• Coagulopathy (INR >1.7, thrombocytopenia <100,000, therapeutic LMWH usage within 24 hours, Thrombin inhibitor use or factor Xa inhibitor use or concomitant abciximab (Reopro)	• Intracranial vascular malformations
	• Concomitant tirofiban (Aggrastat) or eptifibatide (Integrilin)
	• Extra-axial intracranial neoplasms
	• MI within 3 months
• Infective endocarditis	• Acute pericarditis
• Aortic arch dissection	• Cardiac myxoma
• Intra-axial intracranial neoplasm	• Procedural stroke
	• Systemic malignancy
	• Pregnancy if benefit outweighs risk of uterine bleeding
	• Early postpartum period (<14 days)
	• Retinal hemorrhage

GI, gastrointestinal; INR, international normalized ratio; LMWH, low molecular weight heparin; NIHSS, National Institutes of Health Stroke Scale; rtPA, recombinant tissue plasminogen activator.

Table 7.7

Thrombolysis in Cerebral Ischemia Scoring	
Grade 0	No perfusion
Grade 1	Penetration with minimal perfusion
Grade 2	Partial perfusion
– a	Only partial perfusion (2/3) of the entire vascular territory is visualized
– b	Complete filling of all of the expected vascular is visualized, but filling is slower than expected
Grade 3	Complete perfusion

- Seek to identify the cause of the ischemic stroke to implement further management strategies.

Modified Rankin Scale (mRS) is a measure of outcome disability after a stroke. Should be included in the admission history and at 3 months following discharge.

0 No symptoms.
1 No significant disability despite symptoms; able to carry out all ADLs.
2 Slight disability; unable to carry out all activities; able to look after own affairs without assistance.
3 Moderate disability; requires some assistance but able to walk without assistance.
4 Moderately severe disability; unable to wake and attend to bodily needs without assistance.
5 Severe disability; bedridden, incontinent, and requires constant nursing care and attention.
6 Dead.

NEUROIMAGING

CT (or CAT) scans and MRIs are the two most common tests performed on acute neurological conditions. CT scans and especially MRIs can challenge the novice. CT scans emit X-rays towards the patient from a variety of angles, and detectors in the scanner measure the difference between the X-rays absorbed versus transmitted through the body. This difference is referred to as attenuation. The amount of attenuation changes based on the density of the tissue, which is measured in Hounsfield units. High-density tissue, such as bone, absorbs more radiation, thus a reduced amount is detected by the scanner. Low-density tissue, such as the lungs, absorbs less radiation; as such, a greater

Table 7.8

	Color	Hounsfield units
CT Scan Interpretation		
Air	Black	−1,000
Bone	White	1,000
Acute blood	Bright gray	40–70
Chronic blood	Gray	60–100
CSF	Gray	15
Calcification	White	140 to 200
Fat	Dark gray	−50 to −100

signal is detected by the scanner. Attenuation is noted by the difference in color in the images. See Table 7.8 for interpretation of color and Hounsfield units.

MRI interpretation:
MRIs are magnets and create magnetic fields. When a patient is exposed to the strong magnetic field, hydrogen ions align in the direction with the magnetic field. A radiofrequency (RF) pulse is applied and can change the direction and alignment of the hydrogen ions in the body. When the RF pulse is turned off, these ions will then realign with the magnetic field, releasing a signal. The strength of this signal varies between types of tissue (e.g., fat, muscle, water). The MRI machine detects varying ranges of signals from varying planes of magnetization, creating "weighted images." MRIs can also disregard or "suppress" certain signals to create different views of the substances in the resulting pictures. T1 and T2 images highlight different tissues based on the timing of the RF pulses. There are two key differences: In T1, one tissue is bright: fat; whereas in T2, two tissues are bright: fat and water. See Table 7.9 to identify how structures appear on an MRI.

T1 is the most "anatomical" image and can be used to reference anatomical structures or to discriminate between fat and water. Conversely, the cerebrospinal fluid (CSF) is bright in T2 due to increased water content. T2 is generally more commonly used.

In the fluid attenuated inversion recovery (FLAIR) CSF signal is suppressed. This is helpful to evaluate structures in the CNS including the periventricular areas, sulci, and gyri. FLAIR can be used to identify plaques in multiple sclerosis, subtle edema after a stroke, and pathology in other conditions whereby CSF may interfere with interpretation.

Diffusion-weighted imaging (DWI) combines T2 images with the diffusion of water. With DWI view, ischemia can be visualized and can

Table 7.9

Shades of Gray for MRIs

	Bone	CSF	White matter	Gray matter	Fat	Acute blood	Chronic blood	Infarct	Infection
T1	White	Black	White	Gray	White	Gray	White	Dark gray	Dark gray
T2	Bright gray	White	Dark gray	Bright gray	Bright gray	Gray	White	Bright gray	White
FLAIR	Bright gray	Black	Dark gray	Bright gray	Bright gray	Gray	White	Bright gray	White
DWI		Dark gray	Gray	Bright gray		White	White	White	White
SWI		Dark gray	Gray	Bright gray		Black	Black	Black	Black

Acute blood, hours; chronic blood, 1–28 days. DWI, diffusion-weighted images; FLAIR, fluid attenuated inversion recovery; SWI, susceptibility weighted imaging.

detect physiological changes that can happen within minutes (e.g., immediately after a stroke).

Additionally, IV gadolinium contrast can be added to evaluate for thrombosis, vessel dissection, or tumors.

Systematic approach to interpreting MRIs:

- Identify the purpose of each image type to aid in identifying suspected pathology.
  - That is, for a brain MRI, look at T2, then FLAIR, then DWI to help distinguish between most differential diagnoses.
- Verify patient name, date of birth, medical record number, and date of exam.
- Look at the T2 weighted images.
  - Work through the anatomy to assess for abnormal pathology.
  - Compare sides of an image to determine areas of abnormal signaling.
  - Determine shape, size, location, and intensity of the signals.
- Compare different MRI image sequences.
  - Compare T1 to T2 to differentiate between pathologies.
  - View contrast-enhanced images to ascertain vascular pathology.
- Compare against other imaging modalities (e.g., CT scan, plain films).
- Compare against previous MRIs.
  - Are any abnormal signals new or old?
  - Identify changes in the size/shape/brightness of the abnormal signals.
- Consider the clinical context.
  - How unwell is the patient?
  - Are the symptoms acute or chronic?
  - Does the imaged pathology correlate with the presenting symptoms?

DELIRIUM

Causes

D Drugs
E Ears, eyes, or other sensory deficits
L Low O2 (hypoxia)
I Infection, including sepsis
R Restraints, retention (stool or urine)
I Ictal State
U Underhydration, undernutrition
M Metabolic causes (acidosis)

Delirium Prevention

An ounce of prevention is worth a pound of cure is true regarding delirium. Many medication regimens have undergone clinical testing;

Table 7.10

Delirium Prevention Strategies	
Sleep hygiene	• Attempt to keep patient on their usual sleeping schedule. • Allow them to sleep in a recliner if they do so at home.
Minimize noise	• Offer ear plugs. • Turn off TV and music.
Minimize light	• Offer eye masks. • Pull curtains/shades. • Turn down all lights in the room, hallway, and so forth.
Avoid medications	• Including benzodiazepines, anticholinergic agents like diphenhydramine (Benadryl), and other sleep aids (e.g., Ambien).
Cluster care	• Coordinate care, including examinations, at the same time; coordinate with other team members/care teams.
Provide uninterrupted periods of rest	• Space out vital signs to Q 2 or 4 hours as clinically indicated. • Implement quiet-time protocols.

however, no treatment exists to manage delirium. Primary prevention of delirium in all hospitalized patients is paramount (see Table 7.10). Once a patient becomes delirious, the length of stay, cost of care, and risk of death dramatically increase.

PAIN MANAGEMENT

Identifying the type of pain a patient is experiencing is essential to ensuring effective treatment (see Table 7.11). In addition, determining the acuity or chronicity of the pain will provide additional information to understand the acuity or urgency of the situation. Chronic pain is defined as pain that persists for or lasts greater than 3 to 6 months. Many patients have acute and chronic pain simultaneously, which must be addressed separately with separate therapies, with the understanding that therapies will complement each other. Caution must be taken not to cause overmedication, especially in older adults and medically frail persons.

Acute pain management strategies should always include non-pharmacologic strategies along with pharmacologic interventions. Nonpharmacologic strategies commonly include rest, ice, heat, elevation, compression, and stretching. Multimodal pain management strategies should be pursued when prescribing medications for pain management. Multimodal strategies can target multiple receptors, potentiate other treatments, and minimize the use of narcotics. Nonopioid medications include nonsteroidal anti-inflammatory drugs such as ibuprofen

Table 7.11

Types of Pain

	Description	Localization	Example
Neuropathic: • Central or • Peripheral nerves	• Burning • Pins/needles • Tingling • Stabbing • Shooting • Intense • Severe	• Stocking/glove pattern • Radiates down nerve	• Peripheral neuropathy (e.g., diabetes, HIV, chemotherapy) • Neuralgia • Spinal cord or nerve root compression
Somatic: • Skin • Subcutaneous tissue • Joints • Connective tissue • Muscle • Fascia	• Aching • Deep • Cramping • Throbbing • Constant • Dull • Gnawing • Sore • Aching	• Localized • Sometimes radiates to surrounding areas	• Joints • Tendonitis • Bursitis • Gout • Incisional pain • Wounds • Bone • Bone metastasis
Visceral: • Organs • Organ capsule • Connecting structures	• Cramping • Squeezing • Heaviness • Stabbing • Deep • Squeezing • Intense	• Diffuse • Radiates to adjacent or supporting structures	• Angina • Bowel obstruction • Pancreatitis • Cholecystitis

or diclofenac cream, acetaminophen, gabapentin, pregabalin, Lidoderm patch, and epidural catheter with bupivacaine.

Opioids are commonly required to manage acute pain in the surgical and trauma population, as well as among other pain-producing syndromes such as sickle cell crisis, nephrolithiasis, pancreatitis, and so forth. Opioids are highly addictive, thus a plan to wean and stop opioids should be discussed with the patient at the initiation of the agent. Fentanyl, hydromorphone, and morphine are the most commonly prescribed for hospitalized patients. Morphine should be avoided in patients with renal dysfunction, as the metabolites can accumulate, causing overmedication and -sedation.

Older adult patients undergo physiologic changes that make them less sensitive to pain. In addition, changes with the normal aging process and the development and progression of chronic conditions

Table 7.12

Ancillary Tests for Brain Death Testing			
Ancillary test	Date	Time	Results
EEG—Brain death protocol			
Nuclear medicine brain blood flow			
Transcranial Doppler			
Definitive Test:			
4-Vessel cerebral angiography			

Adapted from UMass Memorial Medical Center brain death testing guidelines.

change the pharmacodynamics and pharmacokinetics in the older population. Thus, extreme caution must be used when prescribing pain medications.

Fast Facts

Older patients, especially frail ones, typically can only tolerate very small doses of narcotics. Remember, it's easier to give additional doses than to have to rescue a patient from having been given too much at one time.

BRAIN DEATH

Pronouncement of brain death signifies legal death despite the patient continuing to have a heartbeat (see Table 7.12 and Exhibits 7.1 and 7.2). Cessation of brain function, including the brain stem, requires

- an irreversible and proximate brain injury,
- exclusion of other complicating or confounding medical conditions.
- absence of drug intoxication/poisoning.
- normothermia.
- a period of observation (commonly 24 hours) without clinical improvement, and
- a combination of clinical and ancillary testing:
  - Clinical testing includes absence of brain stem functions and apnea testing.
  - Ancillary tests for adults can include EEG, nuclear scan transcranial Doppler, CT angiogram, and MRI/MRA. Four-vessel cerebral angiography is commonly referred to as a definitive test.

Exhibit 7.1

Sample Brain Death Criteria Template

Prerequisite for clinical diagnosis of brain death:

☐ Known etiology and irreversible conditions:

_____Traumatic brain injury;

_____Subarachnoid hemorrhage

_____Anoxia

_____Other: _____

☐ Head CT results: _____

☐ Core temperature ≥36.0°C

☐ Pulse oximetry ≥90%

☐ Absence of severe hypotension (SBP >100 mmHg for adults)

☐ Absence of severe metabolic abnormalities

☐ Absence of sedatives/CNS depressants, neuromuscular blocking agents, alcohol level <80

Clinical exam:	Results
Date and Time	/
Temperature/HR/BP/O2 Sat	
Absence of cerebral motor response	
Absence of pupillary response to light	
Absence of corneal reflex	
Absence of oculocephalic reflex (doll's eyes)	
Absence of gag reflex	
Absence of oculovestibular reflex (cold calorics)	
Absence of respiratory drive with PaCO2 >60 mmHg or 20 mmHg above patient's baseline	
Examiner's signature/Printed name	/

Adapted from UMass Memorial Medical Center brain death testing guidelines.

Ancillary testing is not always a requirement for brain-death pronouncement, and many societies have their own guidelines. Additionally, each hospital has its own policies and procedures with specific requirements, timeline, and notification of organ procurement centers. Notify the organ procurement center early when a patient has a significant brain injury, or when goals of care discussions are being planned with family.

Some facilities designate specific people who are authorized to perform brain-death testing. Commonly, neurocritical care intensivists, neurologists, neurosurgeons, or other intensivists can declare a patient brain dead. Brain-death testing should not be performed while the patient is in the emergency department.

Exhibit 7.2

Apnea Testing

Apnea testing should be done after confirming absence of brain stem reflexes   Date: Time:

1. Adjust ventilator to normalize PaCO2 (~40 mmHg).*
2. Preoxygenate with 100% FiO2 for 10 minutes.
3. Obtain baseline ABG to establish PaCO2:

   _____/_____/_____/_____
4. Change ventilator to CPAP at 100% FiO2.
5. Observe patient's chest and abdomen for respiration for at least 10 minutes.
6. Draw ABG: to evaluate PaCO2:

   _____/_____/_____/_____

If PaCO2 is >60 mmHg (or >20 mmHg above baseline) and no respiratory effort, patient has confirmed apnea.   PaCO2:   Time:

If PaCO2 is <60 mmHg or <20 mmHg above baseline, continue test and repeat ABG (continue until PaCO2 meets criteria).

If respiratory efforts are observed, apnea is not present; repeat test at a later time.

*For patients with chronic hypercapnia, consider performing a modified apnea test.

DONATION AFTER CARDIAC DEATH (DCD)

The decision to withdraw life-sustaining treatments should be made before and separately from discussion and consideration of donation after cardiac death. This sequencing avoids the perception that patients are being removed from life support to become an organ donor. DCD can be considered if patients are expected to die within close proximity (30 to 60 minutes) of withdrawal of life support. Key tenets to caring for a patient who is a candidate for DCD:

- Separate care teams are required to care for the donor and any potential recipients to avoid a conflict of interest.
- The provider who is caring for the dying patient should pronounce the patient, not the transplant team.
- Discuss specific medications needed to preserve organ function that can be given before death; of which, these medications cannot hasten death.
- Discuss process for consent for procedures needed for organ procurement (e.g., lines, medications)
- A time interval between pronouncement and organ recovery should be predetermined by policy (typically 2 to 5 minutes) to ensure the patient hasn't had spontaneous recovery.

- Be sure that family can be present at the time of death, if they so desire.
- A timeline should be clearly defined when the timeframe between withdrawal of life-sustaining treatments and duration of patient survival precludes organ procurement.

In summary, this chapter reviews anatomy and specific scoring systems for a variety of neurological conditions. The neurological system consistently challenges many NPs, thus having these details at the fingertips can aid in rapid diagnosis and treatment. Frequent review is essential to master neurological content.

References

Claassen, J., Bernardini, G. L., Kreiter, K., Bates, J., Du, Y. E., Copeland, D., Connolly, E. S., & Mayer, S. A. (2001). Effect of cisternal and ventricular blood on risk of delayed cerebral ischemia after subarachnoid hemorrhage: The Fisher scale revisited. *Stroke*, *32*(9), 2012–2020.

Fischer, U., Arnold, M., Nedeltchev, K., Brekenfeld, C., Ballinari, P., Remonda, L., Schroth, G., & Mattle, H. P. (2005). NIHSS score and arteriographic findings in acute ischemic stroke. *Stroke*, *36*(10), 2121–2125.

Fisher, C., Kistler, J., & Davis, J. (1980). Relation of cerebral vasospasm to subarachnoid hemorrhage visualized by computerized tomographic scanning. *Neurosurgery*, *6*(1), 1–9.

Flaherty, J. H., Tariq, S. H., Raghavan, S., Bakshi, S., Moinuddin, A., & Morley, J. E. (2003). A model for managing delirious older inpatients. *Journal of the American Geriatrics Society*, *51*(7), 1031–1035.

Edjlali, M., Rodriguez-Régent, C., Hodel, J., Aboukais, R., Trystram, D., Pruvo, J.-P., Meder, J.-F., Oppenheim, C., Lejeune, J.-P., & Leclerc, X. (2015). Subarachnoid hemorrhage in ten questions. *Diagnostic and Interventional Imaging*, *96*(7–8), 657–666.

Greer, D. M., Shemie, S. D., Lewis, A., Torrance, S., Varelas, P., Goldenberg, F. D., Bernat, J. L., Souter, M., Topcuoglu, M. A., & Alexandrov, A. W. (2020). Determination of brain death/death by neurologic criteria: The World Brain Death Project. *JAMA*, *324*(11), 1078–1097.

Treede, R.-D., Rief, W., Barke, A., Aziz, Q., Bennett, M. I., Benoliel, R., Cohen, M., Evers, S., Finnerup, N. B., & First, M. B. (2015). A classification of chronic pain for ICD-11. *Pain*, *156*(6), 1003.

Moore, D. W. *Neck & Upper Extremity Spine Exam*. www.orthobullets.com/spine/2001/neck-and-upper-extremity-spine-exam

Wiener-Kronish, J. P. (2016). *Handbook of the Massachusetts General Hospital* (6th ed.). Lippincott, Williams & Wilkins.

Hird, R. (2021, 25 February 2021). *The basics of MRI interpretation*. www.geekymedics.com/the-basics-of-mri-interpretation

Kairys, N., Das, J. M., & Garg, M. (2020, 13 October 2020). *Acute Subarachnoid Hemorrhage*. www.ncbi.nlm.nih.gov/books/NBK518975

(2021, 10 November 2018). *Phenytoin correction calculator: Dilantin correction calculator for hypoalbuminemia*. www.clincalc.com/Phenytoin/Correction.aspx?example

Powers, W. J., Rabinstein, A. A., Ackerson, T., Adeoye, O. M., Bambakidis, N. C., Becker, K., Biller, J., Brown, M., Demaerschalk, B. M., & Hoh, B. (2019). Guidelines for the early management of patients with acute ischemic stroke: 2019 update to the 2018 guidelines for the early management of acute ischemic stroke: A guideline for healthcare professionals from the American Heart Association/American Stroke Association. *Stroke, 50*(12), e344–e418.

Powers, W. J., Derdeyn, C. P., Biller, J., Coffey, C. S., Hoh, B. L., Jauch, E. C., Johnston, K. C., Johnston, S. C., Khalessi, A. A., & Kidwell, C. S. (2015). 2015 American Heart Association/American Stroke Association focused update of the 2013 guidelines for the early management of patients with acute ischemic stroke regarding endovascular treatment: A guideline for healthcare professionals from the American Heart Association/American Stroke Association. *Stroke, 46*(10), 3020–3035.

The Joint Commission. (2018). *Modified Rankin Score (mRS)*. https://manual.jointcommission.org/releases/TJC2018A/DataElem0569.html

Rost, N. S., Smith, E. E., Chang, Y., Snider, R. W., Chanderraj, R., Schwab, K., FitzMaurice, E., Wendell, L., Goldstein, J. N., & Greenberg, S. M. (2008). Prediction of functional outcome in patients with primary intracerebral hemorrhage: the FUNC score. *Stroke, 39*(8), 2304–2309.

Hemphill, J. C., Bonovich, D. C., Besmertis, L., Manley, G. T., & Johnston, S. C. (2001). The ICH score. *Stroke, 32*(4), 891–897.

8

Cardiovascular Acute Care

The cardiovascular system is quite expansive, involving numerous diagnoses, diagnostic tests, scoring systems, and treatment regimens, all of which can be challenging to recall. This chapter could not be all inclusive; thus, only selected elements have been included.

In this chapter, you will learn to

- differentiate myocardial ischemia from infarct,
- recognize and treat ST-elevated and non–ST-elevated myocardial infarctions,
- use common vasoactive agents,
- distinguish between shock states,
- differentiate between hypertensive urgency and emergency,
- identify causes of atrial fibrillation, and
- interpret arterial brachial index.

MYOCARDIAL INFARCTIONS

Five distinct types of myocardial infarctions (MI) have been delineated. Documentation of the specific type is required for appropriate billing and classification.

1. Spontaneous: due to acute coronary syndrome (ACS)
2. Non-ACS: ischemic necrosis due to supply/demand imbalance
3. Sudden cardiac death: no biomarkers available

4. Procedural related:

   a. Related to percutaneous intervention (PCI)
   b. Related to stent thrombus

5. Coronary artery bypass graft (CABG)–related

Non–ST-Elevated Myocardial Infarction (NSTEMI)

NSTEMIs have a variety of causes that induce myocardial ischemia, including coronary reasons, noncoronary injury, and increased oxygen demands. Coronary reasons include stable plaque, vasospasm, coronary embolism, and coronary arteritis. Noncoronary causes of NSTEMI include cardiac contusion, myocarditis, and cardiotoxins. Lastly, increased oxygen demands that can lead to NSTEMI include hypotension and all shock states, hypertension, tachycardia, aortic stenosis, and pulmonary embolism. EKG findings that suggest NSTEMI include transient ST elevation, ST depression, and/or new T-wave inversions in more than one lead. Cardiac troponin elevations are noted after 4 hours. Obtain echocardiogram to identify any wall-motion abnormalities, and obtain cardiology consultation.

ST-Elevated Myocardial Infarctions

ST-elevated myocardial infarction (STEMI) is a type 1 MI and is the result of plaque rupture with clot formation in a coronary vessel (see Figures 8.1 and 8.2). The definition of STEMI includes ST segment elevation in two or more contiguous leads ≥2 mm in leads V2 to V3, or ≥1 mm in the other chest leads or limb leads. Activate the STEMI alert within the institution immediately. Obtain echocardiogram to assess cardiac performance, and identify any wall motion or valvular abnormalities (see Table 8.1).

Fast Facts

STEMI definition includes ST segment be elevated in two or more contiguous leads ≥2 mm in leads V2 to V3, or ≥1 mm in the other chest leads or limb leads.

STEMI Treatment

STEMI treatment follows a specific algorithm. Be sure to activate the STEMI alert for your facility to mobilize appropriate resources. For PCI-capable hospitals:

1. Administer aspirin, 325 mg, chewed (buccal absorption).
2. Clopidogrel, 600 mg; or ticagrelor, 180 mg; or prasugrel, 60 mg orally × 1.
3. Heparin, 60 units/kg (maximum 5,000 units), IV bolus.
4. Transfer to cardiac cath lab for primary PCI.

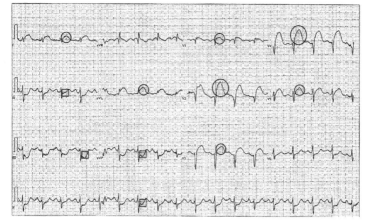

Figure 8.1 ST elevation versus depression.

Key: Box is ST depression; circle is ST elevation.

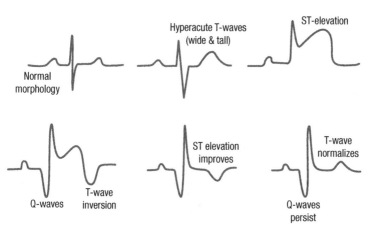

Hyperacute T-waves
(wide & tall)

ST-elevation

Normal
morphology

Q-waves

T-wave
inversion

ST elevation
improves

T-wave
normalizes

Q-waves
persist

Figure 8.2 T-wave progression in STEMI.

For non–PCI-capable hospitals, transfer to PCI facility. If time to PCI will be >120 minutes from first medical contact, consider administration of fibrinolytics:

1. Assess for contraindications to fibrinolytics
   a. Absolute contraindications

      i. Prior intracranial hemorrhage
      ii. Structural cerebral vascular lesions

Table 8.1

12 Lead ECG Leads, Correlating Cardiac Region and Primary Vessel			
I		V1	V4
Lateral	aVR	Septal	Anterior
Cx or Diagonal		LAD	LAD
II	aVL	V2	V5
Inferior	Lateral	Septal	Lateral
RCA	Cx or Diagonal	LAD	Cx or Diagonal
III	aVF	V3	V6
Inferior	Inferior	Anterior	Lateral
RCA > Cx	RCA	LAD	Cx or Diagonal

Cx, circumflex; RCA, right coronary artery; LAD, left anterior descending artery.

    iii. Malignant intracranial neoplasm
    iv. Ischemic stroke in last 90 days
    v. Suspected aortic dissection
    vi. Active bleeding
    vii. Significant traumatic brain injury in last 90 days
    viii. Intracranial or intraspinal surgery within 60 days
    ix. Severe uncontrolled hypertension that is unresponsive to therapy

  b. Relative contraindications

    i. Significant hypertension (SBP >180 or DBP >110)
    ii. Ischemic stroke >3 months
    iii. Dementia
    iv. CPR >10 minutes
    v. Major surgery within 3 weeks
    vi. Recent internal bleeding within 2 to 4 weeks
    vii. Vascular puncture in noncompressible vessel
    viii. Pregnancy
    ix. Active gastric or peptic ulcer
    x. Oral anticoagulant therapy

2. Administer one of the following:

  a. Tenecteplase

    i. Patients <60 kg, administer 30 mg × 1.
    ii. Patients 60 to 69 kg, administer 35 mg × 1.
    iii. Patients 70 to 79 kg, administer 40 mg × 1.
    iv. Patients 80 to 89 kg, administer 45 mg × 1.
    v. Patients >90 kg, administer 50 mg × 1.

b. Reteplase, 10 units IV × 2

c. Alteplase, 15 mg IV × 1, then administer accelerated infusion:

    i. For patients <67 kg, administer .75 mg/kg/dose over 30 minutes, then .5 mg/kg/dose IV over 60 minutes; maximum 100 mg/total dose.

    ii. For patients >67 kg, administer 50 mg over 30 minutes, then 35 mg IV over 60 minutes; maximum 100 mg/total dose.

d. Then follow the previously mentioned STEMI algorithm and arrange transport to PCI facility.

CLINICAL SCORES FOR ACUTE CORONARY SYNDROME (ACS)

A variety of predictor scores have been developed to aid clinicians in the workup of ACS and prioritization of interventions. Use these tools with caution and in conjunction with clinical judgment. Commonly used tools include the TIMI (thrombolysis in Myocardial Infarction) risk score (Table 8.2), HEART (History, ECG, Age, Risk Factors, and Troponin) score (Table 8.3), GRACE (Global Registry of Acute Coronary Events) risk score, HEARTS3 score, and the Hess prediction rule. The HEART score was created specifically for use with emergency department patients.

Table 8.2

TIMI Score and 14-Day Event Rate			
Risk factor	Points	TIMI score	14-day event rate (%)
Age 65–74/≥75	2/3	0–1	4.7
SBP <100	3	2	8.3
HR >100	2	3	13.2
Killip class II to IV	2	4	19.9
Anterior STE or LBBB	1	5	26.2
Diabetes, h/o HTN, or h/o angina	1	6–7	40.9
Weight <67 kg	1		
Time to treatment >4 hours	1		

Scores ranging from 0 to 2 constitute a low risk. Scores of 3–5 are considered intermediate risk. A score of 6 or 7 indicates high risk.

HR, heart rate; HTN, hypertension; LBBB, left bundle branch block; SBP, systolic blood pressure; STE, ST-segment elevation; TIMI, thrombolysis in myocardial infarction.

Table 8.3

The HEART Score for Chest Pain Patients in the ED		
History	– Highly suspicious	– 2 points
	– Moderately suspicious	– 1 point
	– Slightly suspicious or nonspecific	– 0 points
EKG	– Significant ST depression	– 2 points
	– Nonspecific repolarization	– 1 point
	– Normal	– 0 points
Age	– 65 years old	– 2 points
	– 45–65 years old	– 1 point
	– ≤45 years old	– 0 points
Risk factors: HTN, HLD, DM, obesity, current/recent smoker (<1 mo) or FHx of CAD	– >3 factors or FHx of CAD	– 2 points
	– 1 or 2 risk factors	– 1 point
	– 0 risk factors	– 0 points
Troponin	– 3 × normal limit	– 2 points
	– 1 to <3 × normal limit	– 1 point
	– ≤ normal limit	– 0 points

Interpretation: Occurrence of major adverse cardiac events (MACE) at 6 weeks – MACE = AMI, PCI, CABG, and death:
– Score 0–3 = 2.5% MACE over next 6 weeks – discharge home
– Score 4–6 = 30.3% MACE over next 6 weeks – admit for observation
– Score 7–10 = 72.7% MACE over next 6 weeks – early invasive strategies

AMI, acute myocardial infarction; CABG, coronary artery bypass grafting; CAD, coronary artery disease; DM, diabetes mellitus; ED, emergency department; FHx, family history; HLD, hypercholesterolemia; HTN, hypertension; MACE, major adverse cardiac event; PCI, percutaneous coronary intervention.

Thrombolysis in Myocardial Infarction (TIMI) Score

The TIMI score is used to determine the likelihood of ischemic events or mortality in patients with unstable angina or NSTEMI.

Killip Classification

The Killip classification is used with patients who have acute STEMIs to predict inpatient mortality (Table 8.4). The higher the Killip classification, the higher the risk of in-hospital mortality.

HEART FAILURE

A significant sequela of MIs is heart failure, although not all heart failure is caused by MIs or ischemia. AG-ACNPs frequently diagnose and manage heart failure. Ensuring accuracy of terminology, differentiating between left and right heart failure, and identifying the functional classification of heart failure are fundamental skills for AG-ACNPs to possess (see Tables 8.5 to 8.8).

Table 8.4

Killip Classification and Mortality		
Class	Description	Mortality (%)
I	No evidence of CHF	1.5
II	Rales, increased JVD, S3	3.7
III	Pulmonary edema	16.7
IV	Cardiogenic shock	36.7

CHF, congestive heart failure; JVD, jugular venous distention.

Table 8.5

HFpEF vs. HFrEF Comparison		
Classification	Ejection fraction	Description
I. HFrEF	≤40%	Also referred to as systolic heart failure.
II. HFpEF	≥50%	Also referred to as diastolic heart failure.
a. HFmEF	41–49%	HFmEF = heart failure with mid-range ejection fraction. Treatment patterns similar to HFpEF.
b. HFpEF, improved	>40%	Subset of patients with HFpEF previously had HFrEF. Recovery may be clinically different from those with persistently reduced EF.

HFmEF, heart failure mid-range ejection fraction; HFpEF, heart failure with preserved ejection fraction; HFrEF, heart failure with reduced ejection fraction.

Table 8.6

Exam Findings of Right- vs. Left-Sided Heart Failure	
Right	Left
Clinical and Exam Findings: • CVP >15 • Juglar venous distention • Hepatic jugular reflex • Peripheral edema • Pants or shoes fitting tighter	Clinical and Exam Findings: • PCWP >15 • Shortness of breath • Increased work of breathing • Crackles in lung fields • Cephalization on CXR

CVP, central venous pressure; CXR, chest x-ray; PCWP, pulmonary capillary wedge pressure.

SHOCK STATES

Diagnosing and managing shock is central to the AG-ACNP role. Patients who are older, medically frail, and immunocompromised do not always present with classic signs and symptoms, thus diagnosing shock can prove challenging. Additionally, a patient can experience two

Table 8.7

New York Heart Association Functional Classification and Symptom Descriptor

Class	Definition	Other descriptor
I	No symptoms	Asymptomatic
II	Symptoms with ordinary activity	Mild symptoms
III	Symptoms with less-than-ordinary activity	Moderate symptoms
IV	Symptoms at rest or with any minimal activity	Severe symptoms

Table 8.8

ACC/AHA Heart Failure Stages

Stage	Description
A	Patient is at high risk for developing HF in the future but no functional or structural heart disorder.
B	A structural heart disorder but no symptoms.
C	Previous or current symptoms of heart failure in the context of an underlying structural heart problem, managed with medical treatment.
D	Advanced disease requiring hospital-based support, a heart transplant, or palliative care.

ACC, American College of Cardiology; AHA, American Heart Association.

or more types of shock simultaneously. Thus the AG-ACNP must constantly consider and assess for each type of shock (see Table 8.9).

Causes of Hypotension:

C—Cardiac—check EKG and troponin.
H—Hypovolemia—assess fluid status and responsiveness, perform passive leg raise.
A—Anaphylaxis—check recent medications.
S—Sepsis—check lactate.
E—Endocrine—adrenal insufficiency –check random cortisol level.

Shock Index and Modified Shock Index:

Shock index (SI) is defined as the heart rate (HR) divided by systolic blood pressure (SBP) (HR/SBP). Example: HR 110, BP 80/60, SI = 110/80 = 1.375. Normal range is .5 to .7 in healthy adults. A SI >1.1 predicts increased risk for morbidity and mortality, including patients who may need massive transfusion protocol (MTP) activation and/or admission to critical

Table 8.9

Hemodynamics by Type of Shock

Type of shock	CVP/PCWP preload	CO	SVR afterload	SVO2
Hypovolemic	↓	↓	↑	↓
Cardiogenic	↑	↓	↑	↓
Distributive—septic	↓	↑	↓	↑
Distributive—neurogenic	↓	↓	↓	↓
Distributive—anaphylactic	↓	↓	↓	↔
Obstructive	↑	↓	↔	↔
Adrenal insufficiency	↔	↓	↔	↓

CO, cardiac output; CVP, central venous pressure; PCWP, Pulmonary capillary wedge pressure; SVR, systemic vascular resistance.

Table 8.10

Classification of Hemorrhagic Shock

	Class I	Class II	Class III	Class IV
Blood loss	750	750–1,500	1,500–2,000	>2,000
% blood volume	15%	15–30%	30–40%	>40%
HR	<100	>100	>120	>140
BP	Normal	Normal	Decreased	Decreased
Cap refill	Normal	Decreased	Decreased	Decreased
RR	14–20	20–30	30–40	>35
U/O	>30 mL/hr	20–30 mL/hr	5–15 mL/hr	Negligible
Mental status	Slightly anxious	Anxious	Anxious/ confused	Confused/ lethargic
Fluid replacement	Crystalloid	Crystalloid/Blood	Blood	Blood

care units. Alternatively, the modified shock index (MSI) is defined as HR divided by mean blood pressure (MAP), (HR/MAP). Example: HR 110, MAP 50 = MSI = 2.2. An MSI of >1.4 is a predictor of higher morbidity and mortality. The MSI is a stronger predictor of mortality than SI for emergency room patients, as HR and SBP may be influenced by other factors, including pain, agitation, and so forth.

Hemorrhagic shock can be quantified by VS that correlate with amount of hemorrhage (see Table 8.10). Vasoactive agents are commonly required to manage the various types of shock. See Table 8.11 for the variety of vasoactive infusions, dosing, receptor activity, and cardiovascular effects.

Table 8.11

Vasoactive Infusions, Dosing, Receptor Activity, and Cardiovascular Effects

Drug and Doses	Mechanism of action	Main effects
Inopressors		
Dopamine (Inotropin)	β-1+, DA++++	VD+, I++, CH+
.5–5 mcg/kg/min	α+, β-1++, DA+++	VD+, I++++, CH++
5–10 mcg/kg/min	α+++, β-1++, DA+	VC+++, I+++, CH+++,
10–20 mcg/kg/min		HR++, MAP+, CO+
Epinephrine	α+, β-1+++, β-2++	VD+, VC+, I++++, CH++,
.01–.05 mcg/kg/min	α+++, β-1++,	HR+, MAP+, CO++
>.05 mcg/kg/min	β-2++	VC+++, I+++, CH+++,
		HR++, MAP++, CO++
Norepinephrine (Levophed)	α++++, β-1++	VC++++, I+, CH++, HR+-,
.5–30 mcg/min or		MAP+++
.01–.04 mcg/kg/min		
Pure vasopressors		
Angiotensin II (Giapreza)	Angiotensin II	VC+++
.125–40 ng/kg/min		
Phenylephrine	α++++	VC++++, HR Ø/-
(Neosynephrine)		
2–300 mcg/min or		
.1–1 mcg/kg/min		
Vasopressin (Pitressin)	Vasopressin +++	VC++++, MAP+++
.01–.06 units/min		
Inodilators		
Dobutamine (Dobutrex)	α+, β-1++++	VD+, VC+, I+++, CH+,
2–10 mcg/kg/min		HR+, MAP+, CO+
10–20 mcg/kg/min		VD++, VC+, I++++, CH++,
		HR++, MAP v, CO+
Milrinone (Primacor)	cAMP	VD++, I+++, CH+++,
.375–.75 mcg/kg/min		HR++, CO+
Isoproterenol (Isuprel)	β-1++++	VD+, I++++, CH++++,
2–10 mcg/min		HR++++, MAP v, CO+++
Vasodilators		
Nitroglycerine		
1–50 mcg/min	Increases cGMP	Venous vasodilation
>50 mcg/min	production	Arterial vasodilation
Nitroprusside (Nipride)		
10–200 mcg/min	Increases cGMP	Systemic vasodilation
.2–4 mcg/kg/min	production	

CH, chronotropy; CO, cardiac output; HR, heart rate; I, inotropy; MAP, mean arterial blood pressure; Ø, no change; VC, vasoconstriction; VD, vasodilation; +, slight; ++, mild; +++, moderate; ++++, maximum; -, slight decrease; v, variable effects dependent on clinical status.

Medical Sequelae of Shock and Resuscitation:

Patients who experience shock are at high risk for complications. Common complications include ischemia, organ failure, and complications of treatments. Ischemic complications include myocardial ischemia, which may be STEMI or NSTEMIs, ischemic stroke, gastrointestinal ischemia, or deep vein thrombosis. Organ failure includes acute kidney injury/acute renal failure, acute respiratory distress syndrome, and acute liver failure. Sequelae of treatments and interventions include abdominal compartment syndrome, disseminated intravascular coagulation, ventilator-associated pneumonia, and other hospital-acquired infections, with or without multidrug-resistant organisms, multisystem organ failure, pressure ulcers, ICU-acquired weakness from critical illness myopathy or neuropathy, and post-ICU syndrome. The AG-ACNP must maintain a high index of suspicion to identify these sequelae. Additionally, the AG-ACNP should institute preventative measures and undertake ongoing assessment and monitoring for early identification and treatment of such complications.

SEVERE HYPERTENSION VERSUS HYPERTENSIVE EMERGENCY

The primary factor distinguishing between hypertensive urgency and emergency is target organ damage. Should a patient develop encephalopathy, acute kidney injury, MI, aortic dissection, and so forth, then hypertensive emergency is diagnosed. Both conditions require controlled reduction in blood pressure to prevent further injury to organs (see Table 8.12 for medication infusions and dosing). Identifying the causative factor is critical to prevent relapse. Commonly, the causative factor is decreased medication adherence, which requires further exploration. Assess for cost increases; prescription not being refilled in a timely manner; patient unable to pick up prescription from pharmacy or prescription not delivered in a timely manner; insurance changes requiring preauthorization or change to a higher-tier copay; or that the patient confused medications or could not tolerate side effects. Be sure to engage social work and case management along with primary care provider (PCP) to identify cost-effective treatment options prior to discharge.

Fast Facts

Hypertensive emergency should have blood pressure reductions of no greater than 25% in the first 24 hours to prevent hypoperfusion of vital organs, which could cause further target organ damage.

Table 8.12

IV Antihypertensive Infusions and/or Bolus Dosing

Drug	MOA	Dosing
Diltiazem (Cardizem)	Non-dihydropyridine calcium channel blocker	Initial bolus 2.5–10 mg followed by an infusion 2.5–15 mg/hr
Esmolol (Breviblock)	Selective beta-1 blocker	Initial bolus of 50 mcg, followed by an infusion 50–300 mcg/kg/min
Labetalol (Trandate)	Selective alpha-1 and nonselective beta-1 and beta-2 blocker	20–80 mg IV Q 10–30 min, or 1–2 mg/min IV infusion
Nicardipine (Cardene)	Dihydropyridine calcium channel blocker	Infusion: 5 mg/hr IV, may increase by 2.5 mg/hr Q 5–15 min to max of 15 mg/hr
Enalapril (Vasotec)	Angiotensin-converting enzyme inhibitor	1.25 mg IV Q 6 hr; max 20 mg/24 hr; avoid or reduce dose in acute kidney injury **Fetal/neonatal morbidity/mortality, d/c drug ASAP when pregnancy detected.
Nitroprusside (Nipride)	Vasodilator/nitrate	3–4 mcg/kg/min IN infusion; increase by .5 mcg/kg/min Q 5 min max 10 mcg/kg/min **Cyanide and thiocyanate metabolites can be toxic at higher levels.

ATRIAL FIBRILLATION

Atrial fibrillation (AF) is a common problem for AG-ACNPs to diagnose and manage. Determine whether this is an existing or new problem. New AF must be evaluated and causative factor(s) determined in order to treat appropriately. An easy mnemonic to recall causes of AF is PIRATES.

Causes of atrial fibrillation:

P—Pulmonary embolism, potassium
I—Ischemia, infection, inflammation
R—Respiratory distress
A—Atrial enlargement = volume overload
T—Thyroid disease
E—Ethanol intake
S—Sepsis, sleep apnea

Fast Facts

Identifying the cause of AF is key to effective treatment.

Table 8.13

CHA₂DS₂VASC Score

Risk factor	Score	Risk factor	Score
CHF or LVEF ≤40%	1	Stroke/TIA/Thromboembolism	2
Hypertension	1	Vascular disease	1
Age ≥75	2	Age 65–74	1
Diabetes	1	Female	1
Interpretation: CHEST 2018		Interpretation: AHA/ACC/HRS 2019	
– 1 for males or – 2 for females – (i.e., at least one non-sex risk factor)		– 2 for males or – 3 for females – (i.e., at least two non-sex risk factors)	
First line therapy (for both) is DOAC therapy over warfarin.			

ACC, American College of Cardiology; AHA, American Heart Association; CHF, congestive heart failure; DOAC, direct oral anticoagulant; HRS, Heart Rhythm Society; LVEF, left ventricular ejection fraction; TIA, transient ischemic attack.

Fast Facts

Carotid massage is no longer an acceptable vagal maneuver for atrial fibrillation due to the high risk of carotid artery plaque rupture, causing embolic ischemic strokes.

The decision to anticoagulate hospitalized patients with AF is complicated, and many factors should be considered, including the cause of AF, the duration of AF, and a comparison of the risks of stroke versus bleeding. Comparing the results of the CHA₂DS₂VASC score and the HAS-BLED scores to see which is greater will aid discussions with the patient and their family (see Tables 8.13 and 8.14).

VASCULAR DISORDERS

Aneurysms

Three types of aortic aneurysms exist, including ascending thoracic, descending thoracic, and abdominal aneurysms. Thoracic aortic aneurysms are commonly asymptomatic, with many being detected incidentally during other diagnostic testing of the chest. Risk factors include hypertension, connective tissue disorders such as Marfan syndrome or Ehlers-Danlos, bicuspid aortic valve, massive blunt chest trauma, cocaine

Table 8.14

HAS-BLED Score and Interpretation

Risk factor	Score
Hypertension (SBP >160)	1
Abnormal renal or liver function	1–2
Stroke	1
Bleeding tendency or predisposition	1
Labile INR	1
Age >65	1
Drugs (concomitant ASA/NSAIDs) or alcohol	1–2

Interpretation: 0–2 = low risk of bleeding; ≥3 = high risk of bleeding.

ASA, aspirin; INR, international normalized ratio; NSAIDS, nonsteroidal anti-inflammatory drug; SBP, systolic blood pressure.

abuse, and preeclampsia. Symptoms are a result of compressed anatomy as the aneurysm expands. Symptoms include shortness of breath, wheezing, dysphagia, and hoarseness. Mediastinal widening on chest X-ray and associated murmur of aortic regurgitation due to involvement of the bicuspid aortic valve are common exam findings. Indications for repair include symptomatic aneurysms and aneurysms over 5.5 cm in diameter for the general population, and 5.0 cm in those with bicuspid aortic valve. The Stanford classification denotes two types of aneurysms. Type A aneurysms extend from the aortic root through the aortic arch, and type B aneurysms extend along the descending aorta.

Abdominal aneurysms are defined as dilatation of the aorta ≥3 cm. Screening abdominal ultrasounds are recommended for all men ages 65 to 75 with any smoking history. Rupture is more common with aneurysms ≥5 cm and pose a 12% mortality for men and 18% for women, which increases dramatically as the aneurysm increases in size.

Aortic dissections commonly present with the patient complaining of sudden severe back pain or syncope. The pain is classically described as tearing or ripping in nature but more commonly as sharp or stabbing. An exam can reveal unequal pulses or pulse deficits in approximately 30% of patients. Computerized tomography angiography (CTA) scans are the gold standard for diagnosing aortic dissections.

Preoperative management and medical management for nonsurgical candidates include aggressive blood pressure management. IV labetalol prn or labetalol or esmolol infusions to achieve systolic blood pressure <120 mmHg and a heart rate close to 60 beats per minute. Definitive surgical intervention is essential, as every hour delay substantially increases mortality. Endovascular repair is the recommended approach for repair.

Complications of aneurysms and their associated dissection or rupture include acute kidney injury, ischemic stroke, spinal cord ischemia, postoperative hemorrhage, and mesenteric ischemia. Mesenteric ischemia is rare but has significant mortality, and is manifested by persistent lactic acidosis or bowel movements early in the postoperative period.

Fast Facts

Preoperative goals for aortic dissections are systolic blood pressure <120 mmHg and a heart rate of 60 beats per minute. Aggressively titrate labetalol or esmolol infusions to urgently achieve these goals.

Venous Thromboembolism

Venous thromboembolism (VTE) and peripheral arterial disease (PAD) are common conditions AG-ACNPs will diagnose and manage. While differentiating between the pathophysiology of these two phenomena seems logical, many students and new NPs can get confused. Especially important to consider are the consequences of deep vein thrombosis (DVT) migrating and becoming a pulmonary embolus (PE) and risk factors of PAD progressing to acute limb ischemia, both of which could lead to loss of limb or life (see Table 8.15).

Every hospitalized patient should have DVT prophylaxis ordered upon admission. Both mechanical and chemoprophylaxis should be ordered unless contraindicated. If contraindications are present, they must be documented. Failure to document contraindications leads legal experts to contend it was negligence on the provider's part should an ill-intended consequence occur. Additionally, early mobility is critical for DVT prevention as well as for other benefits.

To determine the patient's probability of having a DVT, calculate the Wells Criteria score. For moderate or high suspicion for DVT, consider additional diagnostic testing based on the likelihood of the patient having a DVT (see Table 8.16).

Diagnostic Testing

D-dimer has about 98% sensitivity but only 50% specificity and is useful to rule out VTE/PE; however, it is not recommended for use in patients who already have their coagulation cascade triggered, such as surgical or trauma patients, or cancer or pregnant patients. Venous duplex is the best test to diagnose DVT. CT angiogram is indicated when pulmonary embolus (PE) is suspected. When patients are too unstable hemodynamically or contrast load is contraindicated, consider transthoracic echocardiogram (TTE). TTE can demonstrate right ventricular strain, or dysfunction, but is not diagnostic for PE.

Table 8.15

Comparison of DVT and PAD Risk Factors and Symptomatology

Deep vein thrombosis	Peripheral arterial disease
Risk factors	Risk factors
– Major surgery or trauma (abdominal, pelvic, hip/knee replacement)	– Atrial fibrillation
– Cancer	– Hyperlipidemia
– Immobility	– Diabetes
– Pregnancy	– Smoking
– Obesity	– Medications (COX-2 inhibitors)
– Contraceptive use or hormone replacement	– Devices (mechanical valve)
– Invasive devices (PICC lines, CVC)	– Aneurysms with distal embolization
– Heparin-induced thrombocytopenia	– External compression
– Hereditary factors (Factor V Leiden deficiency, antithrombin deficiency, protein C deficiency, protein S deficiency, antiphospholipid syndrome)	– History of prior trauma
	– Vasculitis
	– Radiation injury
Signs and Symptoms	Signs and Symptoms
– Pain (mild)/tenderness	– Claudication
– Unilateral edema of affected leg/foot, may be bilateral edema if DVT is bilateral	– Pale
	– Poor nail/hair growth
– Erythema	– Cooler extremity
– Warmth	– Thin, shiny skin
– Change in color	– Reduced ankle-brachial index

CVC, central venous catheter; DVT, deep vein thrombosis; PAD, peripheral arterial disease; PICC, peripherally inserted central catheter.

The primary treatment option for most patients is systemic anticoagulation. Refer to the American College of Chest Physicians (ACCP) guidelines for VTE treatment. Medication options include unfractionated heparin, low-molecular-weight heparin, and oral anticoagulants. For patients who have contraindications to systemic anticoagulation, consider a temporary inferior vena cava (IVC) filter. For patients with RV strain or hemodynamic instability, consider systemic thrombolytic therapy (alteplase 100 mg IV over 2 hours) or catheter-directed thrombolysis. Consult interventional radiology or vascular surgery for endovascular thrombectomy. Extracorporeal membrane oxygenation (ECMO) may be required to bridge patient to an open surgical thrombectomy by a cardiothoracic surgeon. Assess whether or not your institution has a pulmonary embolism response team and how to access them, prior to an emergent situation.

Table 8.16

Simplified Wells Criteria for DVT	
Clinical indicator:	**Points**
Active cancer (ongoing treatment or within 6 months)	1
Paralysis or recent immobilization of lower extremity	1
Recent bed rest for ≥3 days or major surgery within 3 months	1
Local tenderness along deep vein system	1
Entire leg swelling	1
Calf ≥3 cm larger (at 10 cm below tibial tuberosity)	1
Pitting edema of affected leg	1
Collateral superficial veins (nonvaricose)	1
Previous DVT	1
Alternative diagnosis at least as likely	−2

Pretest probability:		
Score 0	Score 1 or 2	Score >3
Low probability (5%)	Moderate (17%)	High probability (53%)

DVT, deep vein thrombosis.

Limb Ischemia

PAD can lead to chronic or acute limb ischemia. Modification of risk factors can stop the progression of atherosclerosis and its associated sequelae. Monitor ankle brachial indexes for progression of chronic limb ischemia. Ankle brachial indexes of .41 to .9 are typical for patients complaining of claudication. Critical limb ischemia is denoted with an ABI <.41 and requires referral to a vascular surgeon, if this has not been done previously.

Ankle-Brachial Index

The ankle-brachial index (ABI) is the systolic pressure of the posterior tibial artery divided by the highest systolic blood pressure of either brachial artery. The ABI is both a sensitive and specific metric to diagnose PAD. Segmental blood pressures in the thigh, calf, ankle, and metatarsal regions can help pinpoint the blockage. Interpretation of ABIs is noted in Table 8.17.

Acute Limb Ischemia

Acute limb ischemia is a surgical emergency, occurring when arterial blood flow is completely disrupted to an extremity. The hallmark sign

Table 8.17

ABI Interpretation		
ABI value	Interpretation	Action
>1.4	Calcified or hardened vessel, noncompressible	Refer to vascular surgeon
1.0–1.4	Normal	Modify risk factors
.9–1.0	Acceptable	Modify risk factors
.8–.9	Some arterial disease	Modify risk factors
.5–.8	Moderate arterial disease	Refer to vascular surgeon
<.5	Severe arterial disease	Refer to vascular surgeon

is abrupt onset of excruciating pain in the affected limb. Additionally, patients commonly complain of numbness or paresthesia and paralysis. Pulses are absent and the limb is cool to touch. Anticoagulation and either open or endovascular reperfusion interventions are the immediate interventions required to salvage the limb.

Fast Facts

Classic signs of acute limb ischemia include the six Ps: pain, pallor, paresthesia, paralysis, pulselessness, and poikilothermia (cool to touch).

In summary, this chapter summarizes a small fragment of required knowledge for AG-ACNPs to care for patients with cardiovascular disease. The most lethal or limb-threatening problems have been touched upon. Be sure to do in-depth reading of texts and clinical practice guidelines to support your knowledge base.

References

Aday, A. W., & Beckman, J. A. (2017). Diseases of the Aorta. In S. C. McKean, J. J. Ross, D. D. Dressler, & D. B. Scheurer (Eds.), *Principles and Practice of Hospital Medicine* (2nd ed., pp. 2107–2114). McGraw Hill Education.

Basit, H., Malik, A., & Huecker, M. R. (2021). *Non ST segment elevation myocardial infarction*. StatPearls Publishing. www.ncbi.nlm.nih.gov/books/NBK513228

Casey, S., Lanting, S., Oldmeadow, C., & Chuter, V. (2019). The reliability of the ankle brachial index: A systematic review. *Journal of Foot and Ankle Research*, *12*(1), 39. https://doi.org/10.1186/s13047-019-0350-1

Kearon, C., Akl, E. A., Ornelas, J., Blaivas, A., Jimenez, D., Bounameaux, H., Huisman, M., King, C. S., Morris, T. A., Sood, N., Stevens, S. M., Vintch, J. R. E., Wells, P., Woller, S. C., & Moores, L. (2016). Antithrombotic therapy for VTE disease: CHEST guideline and expert panel report. *Chest, 149*(2), 315–352. https://doi.org/10.1016/j.chest.2015.11.026

Koch, E., Lovett, S., Nghiem, T., Riggs, R. A., & Rech, M. A. (2019). Shock index in the emergency department: Utility and limitations. *Open Access Emergency Medicine,* 179–199. https://doi.org/10.2147/OAEM.S178358

Lawler, P. R., & Morrow D. A. (2017). Cardiovascular conditions in the ICU —Acute Coronary syndromes and other common cardiac problems. In G. Frendl & R. D. Urman (Eds.), *Pocket ICU* (2nd ed., pp. 1–15). Wolters Kluwer.

McDaniel, M. (2017). Acute coronary syndromes. In S. J. McKean, J. J. Ross, D. D. Dressler, & D. B. Scheurer (Eds.), *Principles and Practice of Hospital Medicine* (2nd ed., pp. 929–940). McGraw Hill Education.

Mekkaoui, S., Pelletier-Bui, A., & Ginty, C. (2017, 18 April 2017). *Back to basics: ECG findings in acute myocardial infarction: Identifying the culprit vessel.* www.emdaily.cooperhealth.org/content/back-basics-ecg-findings-acute-myocardial-infarction-identifying-culprit-vessel

Palmer, L. J. & Berg, S. (2017). Vascular surgical critical care. In G. Frendl & R. D. Urman (Eds.), *Pocket ICU* (pp. 1–4). Wolters Kluwer.

Shah, S. K., & Belkin, M. (2017). Acute and chronic lower limb ischemia. In S. J. McKean, J. J. Ross, D. D. Dressler, & D. B. Scheurer (Eds.), *Principles and Practice of Hospital Medicine* (pp. 211–212). McGraw Hill Education.

Wever-Pinzon, O. & Fang, J. C. (2017). Heart failure. In S. J. McKean, J. J. Ross, D. D. Dressler, & D. B. Scheurer (Eds.), *Principles and Practice of Hospital Medicine* (2nd ed., pp. 941–953). McGraw Hill Education.

9

Pulmonary Acute Care

Acutely and critically ill hospitalized patients are frequently admitted with or develop acute hypoxic and/or hypercarbic respiratory failure. AG-ACNPs must be adept at managing acute respiratory decompensation, including deciding when to intubate versus manage with noninvasive ventilation. Managing, weaning, and troubleshooting ventilators are essential skills for AG-ACNPs even when working outside the ICU, as an ICU bed may not be readily available. Rapid diagnosis and treatment of acute respiratory disorders can be lifesaving, whereas failure to rescue can have serious repercussions. Frequent reassessment is required minutes, hours, and days after extubation so as to intervene early to prevent reintubation.

In this chapter, you will learn

- airway management,
- ventilator management and extubation criteria,
- management of asthma exacerbation,
- a stepwise process to interpret chest x-rays, and
- to differentiate between exudative and transudative pleural effusions.

AG-ACNPs will routinely diagnose and manage patients who develop acute and/or chronic hypoxic and/or hypercarbic respiratory failure. Respiratory failure is one of the most common conditions requiring a rapid-response team and admission to the ICU. Astute assessment, appropriate diagnostics, accurate diagnosis of the cause of respiratory failure, and focused interventions can prevent intubation, which in turn can prevent medical sequelae of mechanical ventilation. The AG-ACNP must be able to differentiate between hypoxic and

Table 9.1

Acute Respiratory Failure	
Hypoxic	**Hypercarbic**
Also known as type I respiratory failure PaO_2 <60 mmHg	Also known as type II respiratory failure $PaCO_2$ >45
Causes: • Right-to-left shunt • V/Q mismatch • Alveolar hypoventilation • Diffusion defect • Inadequate O_2	Causes: • Muscular weakness • Increased CO_2 production • Right-to-left shunt • Increased dead space
Examples: • Pulmonary edema • Pneumonia • Acute lung injury • Atelectasis • Aspiration • Pulmonary contusion • Acute pneumonitis • Pulmonary embolism	Examples: Neuromuscular causes: • DNS depression • Brainstem injury • Spinal cord injury • Neuropathy • Neuromuscular junction • Myopathy • Kyphoscoliosis Pulmonary causes: • COPD • Asthma • Cystic fibrosis • Bronchiectasis

COPD, chronic obstructive pulmonary disease; DNS, dynamic neuromuscular stabilization.

hypercarbic respiratory failure, as the causative factors and interventions are divergent (see Table 9.1).

AIRWAY MANAGEMENT

Noninvasive Positive Pressure Ventilation

Patients with acute hypoxic and/or hypercarbic respiratory failure caused by processes that can resolve within 48 hours can be trialed on noninvasive positive pressure ventilation (NPPV). Continuous positive airway pressure (CPAP) is used predominantly for acute hypoxic respiratory failure without hypercarbia. Bilevel positive pressure airway pressure (BiPAP) is used for hypercarbic respiratory failure with or without hypoxia. The additional inspiratory pressure of BiPAP causes augmented tidal volumes, thus increasing minute ventilation and thus blowing off carbon dioxide. Conditions that preclude use of NPPV include:

- cardiac or respiratory arrest
- unstable hemodynamics
- altered mental status without ability to protect airway
- inability to effectively manage airway or oral secretions
- large amounts of pulmonary secretions
- abnormal anatomy or airway
- traumatic facial or neck injuries with significant bleeding or risk of edema
- inability to remove mask if the patient were to vomit
- recent esophageal surgery

Intubation

Many AG-ACNPs who work at nonteaching hospitals will be credentialed to intubate at their respective facility. Others who work at academic or teaching centers with anesthesia residencies will not need to intubate, as that skill is part of the resident's learning process. Regardless, the NP plays a vital role in deciding when to intubate, assessing risk factors for difficult intubations, mobilizing resources, coordinating team members, and managing the patient during this high-risk period. The NP is responsible for monitoring vital signs during the procedure, communicating with the intubating provider when O2 saturation drops or bradycardia occurs, and is responsible for stabilizing the heart rate and responding to hypotension.

Indications for Intubation:

- Depressed mental status and inability to protect the airway (lack of cough or gag reflexes)
- Severe pulmonary, facial, neck, or multisystem trauma
- Airway edema (burns, anaphylaxis, epiglottitis, infection, obstructing mass)
- Need for secretion management/airway clearance
- Tachypnea >35 breaths per minute
- Hypoxia refractory to maximized oxygen delivery
- Hypercarbic respiratory failure refractory to NPPV
- Minimize oxygen consumption and maximize oxygen delivery (sepsis/shock)
- Need for procedural sedation in setting of tenuous airway
- To obtain critical imaging
- Temperature control (serotonin syndrome)

Mallampati Score

The Mallampati score is used to identify patients who are at risk for difficult endotracheal intubation (see Figure 9.1). The classification is a universal language to describe anatomic qualities of the airway when a patient opens their mouth and sticks out their tongue. Scores range from 1 to 4; with a score of 4, the tongue fully obscures the soft palate.

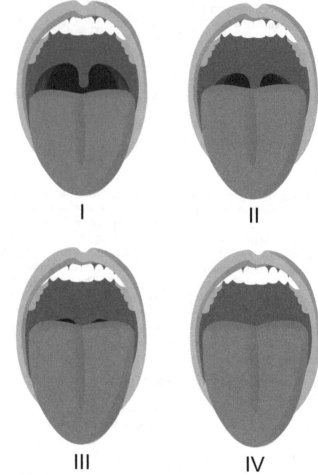

Figure 9.1   Mallampati score.

Cormack-Lehane Airway Grading

This scoring system describes the view of the vocal chords under direct laryngoscope. Scores range from 1 to 4; with higher numbers, the poorer the view of the vocal chords, the more difficult the intubation. For grades 3 and 4, adjunct intubation equipment should be readily available.

Difficult Airway

Patients with known difficult airways should have notation of this easily identifiable in their chart and in their room/door way. A GlideScope, fiberoptic bronchoscope, subglottic airway device, bougie or tube exchanger, cricothyrotomy kit, and tracheostomy kit should all be readily available for difficult airways. In nonemergent situations, early notification of the anesthesia team and surgical team is essential for successful planning of airway insertion.

AG-ACNP's Role

As the AG-ACNP managing a patient with a difficult airway, defer intubation to an expert team. Early and advanced notice of an impending intubation is helpful to the airway team. Have previous intubation notes open and ready for review by the airway team. Ensure that the patient has adequate IV access for administration of medications. Prescribe intubation medications if the airway team doesn't bring their own. Additionally, prescribe postintubation sedation and analgesics.

During the intubation, you may be called upon to administer induction medications, provide cricoid pressure, manually ventilate with the Ambu bag, or call for additional backup. Additionally, if the patient is not currently in an intensive care unit (ICU) at the time of intubation, the AG-ACNP should initiate transfer to the ICU as soon as possible. The AG-ACNP can delegate this first step to a charge nurse or house supervisor. A delay in notification can result in a delay in transfer, as ICU beds may not be readily available.

Anticipate hypotension. Remember, the patient may have a significant amount of adrenaline circulating due to their increased work of breathing, anxiety, hypoxia, and so forth. Once sedation is given, the patient will relax and sedatives will further reduce blood pressure. Thus, ensure that a bolus of fluid is connected to the patient's IV. Have vasopressors ready and have a low threshold to initiate if an IV fluid bolus is insufficient to maintain mean arterial blood pressure above 65 mmHg.

Anticipate the worst-case scenario. Patients may have arrhythmias and/or cardiac arrest during intubation. Consider the reasons for the cardiac arrest, which is commonly related to hypoxia or hypotension. First, ensure that the endotracheal tube is in good position. Ensure adequate oxygenation/ventilation, and follow advanced cardiac life support (ACLS) algorithms.

Post-Intubation Care

Immediately after intubation, the AG-ACNP should assess endotracheal tube (ETT) position. Auscultate breath sounds bilaterally and over epigastric area. Then confirm with end tidal carbon dioxide (etCO2) monitoring, and then finally with a chest x-ray (see Tables 9.2 and 9.3) to ensure placement of the ETT below the bottom of the clavicles and 2 cm above the carina. Additionally, assess for pneumothorax, placement of an orogastric tube, and/or placement of a central venous catheter if inserted prior to obtaining a chest x-ray.

Table 9.2

Color of Tissues on X-rays	
Black	Air
Dark gray	Fat
Gray	Soft tissue
Bright gray	Bone
Bright white	Metal

https://undergradimaging.pressbooks.com/chapter/x-rays

Table 9.3

Tips for Interpretation of Chest X-rays	
Quality of the Film—I RIP ABCDEFGHI	
I = Identification	Do you have the right patient and the right date? Does this look like the correct patient?
R = Rotation	Confirm equal distance between medial ends of clavicles and vertebral spinous process.
I = Inspiration	Good inspiration is if 9 posterior (or 6 anterior) ribs are visible above the mid-diaphragm.
P = Penetration	The radiograph is adequately penetrated if vertebral bodies are just visible through the cardiac shadow.
Assessment for Pathology	
A = Airway	Is the trachea midline between the ends of the clavicles? Any deviations?
B = Bones	Assess for any fractures, and assess the quality of the bones.
C = Cardiac silhouette	Review heart size (PA film less than half the diameter of the thorax), assess position, borders, shape.
D = Diaphragm	Assess costophrenic and cardiophrenic angles, assess for pleural effusions, atelectasis, elevations, flattening.
E = Edges and external soft tissue	Assess edges for pneumothorax. Look at the external soft tissues for subcutaneous air. Assess soft tissues for foreign bodies, implants.
F = Fields	Assess lung fields. Compare sides for differences in density. Assess lung fissures, vascularity, nodules, consolidation, and masses.
G = Gastric bubble	Inspect for lucency in upper-left quadrant. Any overdistention of air?
H = Hilum	Assess for widened mediastinum. Any aortic or tracheal calcifications?

(continued)

Table 9.3

Tips for Interpretation of Chest X-rays (*continued*)	
I = Insertions	Check for inserted devices (e.g., tubes, lines, and drains), endotracheal or tracheostomy tubes, nasogastric tubes, central lines, ports or PICC lines, chest tubes, pacemakers, AICDs, or other medical equipment.

AICDs, automatic implantable cardiac defibrillators; PICC, peripherally inserted central venous catheters.

Fast Facts

Upon intubation, the AG-ACNP should personally assess bilateral lung sounds, auscultate the epigastric area, observe for end tidal CO2 level, and assess the position of the endotracheal tube on the CXR.

Ventilator Management

AG-ACNPs must be prepared to manage ventilators regardless whether the AG-ANCP works in an ICU or not. ICU beds are in high demand and may not be readily available. Thus, the AG-ACNP in the ED, rapid-response teams, in postanesthesia care units, on the hospitalist or specialty services may be required to manage intubated patients until an ICU bed becomes available.

Initial Ventilator Settings

Step 1: Calculate ideal body weight (IBW).
  For men, start at 50 kg and add 2.2 kg for each inch over 5 feet.
  For women, start at 45 kg and add 2.2 kg for each inch over 5 feet.
  Note: Be sure to use a tape measure to obtain an actual height.
Step 2: Select a mode of ventilation. Names of specific ventilation modes vary by manufacturer (see Tables 9.4, 9.5, and 9.6).
  A generic nomenclature has been developed to standardize concepts. The nomenclature has three elements (see Figure 9.2).
Step 3: Select a tidal volume to either set or limit—initially should be ≤8 mL/kg IBW; for adult respiratory distress syndrome (ARDS), should be ≤6 mL/kg IBW.
Step 4: Set rate—initially try to match the patient's respiratory rate to minimize the work of breathing.
Step 5: Set FiO2—always good for patients who are newly intubated for hypoxic respiratory failure to start at 100% and can wean rapidly if O2 saturations remain >93%.
Step 6: Select PEEP level—minimal PEEP level is 5; for obese and morbidly obese patients, PEEP is minimally 7.5 mmH2O. Prior to

Table 9.4

Ventilator Modes		
Preferred term	**Intended meaning mechanical ventilation with …**	**Old terminology—avoid**
Volume-controlled continuous mandatory ventilation (VC-CMV)	Preset TV and inspiratory flow. Every breath is mandatory (i.e., inspiration is patient or machine triggered and machine cycled).	Assist/control, A/C, CMV, volume assist/control, volume-limited ventilation, volume-controlled ventilation, controlled ventilation, volume-targeted ventilation
Volume-controlled intermittent mandatory ventilation (VC-IMV)	Preset TV and inspiratory flow. Spontaneous breaths can exist between mandatory breaths.	Synchronized intermittent mandatory ventilation (SIMV)
Pressure-controlled continuous mandatory ventilation (PC-CMV)	Present inspiratory pressure and inspiratory time. Every breath is mandatory.	Assist/control, A/C, CMV, pressure assist/control, pressure control, pressure-limited ventilation, pressure-controlled ventilation, pressure-targeted ventilation
Pressure-controlled intermittent mandatory ventilation (PC-IMV)	Preset inspiratory pressure and inspiratory time. Spontaneous breaths can exist between mandatory breaths.	Synchronized intermittent mandatory ventilation (SIMV)
Continuous spontaneous ventilation (CSV)	Any mode of mechanical ventilation where every breath is spontaneous.	Spontaneous

Table 9.5

Ventilator Terminology	
Terminology	**Definition**
Mandatory breath	A type of breath that is machine triggered and cycled
Spontaneous breath	A type of breath that is patient triggered and cycled
Assisted breath	A type of breath that is supported in part by the ventilator
Patient-triggered breath	A breath that is triggered by the patient, independent of ventilator settings or frequency
Auto-triggering	Unintended triggering of the ventilator to deliver a breath (i.e., from an external source or inappropriate trigger sensitivity)

Table 9.6

Pros and Cons of Each Mode of Ventilation

Mode	Pros	Cons	Major settings	Monitor
Continuous spontaneous ventilation (CSV)	Used as a weaning mode; most comfortable	No guaranteed rate or ventilation; patient can fatigue	FiO2, PEEP	TV, MV
Volume-controlled intermittent mandatory ventilation (VC-IMV)	Can be a weaning mode or for relatively healthy people (e.g., post-op elective surgery)		TV, RR, FiO2 PEEP	Spontaneous TV and RR; PIP/plateau pressures on ventilated breaths
Volume control (VC)	Ensures minimum minute ventilation	Monitor peak/plateau pressures to avoid barotrauma	TV, RR, FiO2, PEEP	PIP/plateau pressures
Pressure-controlled continuous mandatory ventilation (PC-CMV)	Limits pressure to avoid barotrauma	At risk for low or high TV; monitor to avoid volutrauma or hypoventilation	Inspiratory pressure, RR, FiO2, PEEP	TV, MV
Pressure-regulated volume control (PRVC)	Guarantees TV but delivers pressure-controlled breaths	At risk for low or high pressure	Targeted TV, RR, O2, PEEP	Pressures and volumes
Airway pressure release ventilation (APRV)	Good for ARDS patients who are spontaneously breathing	Complex mode/settings, risk of lung injury if set improperly	Time high, time low, PEEP high, PEEP low, FiO2	Volumes, CO2 exchange

and during intubation, patients will derecruit alveoli; thus, start with a higher PEEP levels of 10 mmHg will rerecruit alveoli and improve hypoxia. Wean PEEP after FiO2 is ≤50%.

Step 7: Obtain ABG and adjust settings based on ABG.

Arterial blood gas interpretation can be found in Chapter 10. To adjust the PaCO2, adjust the TV or rate. Hypercarbia contributes to respiratory

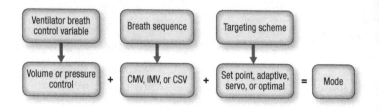

Figure 9.2   Standard nomenclature for ventilators.

acidosis, whereas low PaCO2 creates an alkalotic state. Oxygen does not cleave off hemoglobin in an alkalotic state, thus causing further cellular hypoxia.

To adjust the PaO2, adjust the FiO2 or PEEP.

Step 8: Continue to monitor peak inspiratory pressure (PIP) and plateau pressures.

- PIP reflects the amount of pressure required for the ventilator to deliver each breath. Normal PIP is <40 cm H2O; varies depending on resistance (i.e., patient coughing or biting on tube, size of tube, secretions in tube).
- Plateau pressure reflects the amount of pressure remaining in the lungs when inspiration ceases; goal plateau pressure is <30 cm H2O. Trend plateau pressures–keep <30 cmH2O pressure. If trending up or above, then TV needs to be increased.

Ventilator Weaning and Extubation Criteria

Every ventilated patient should have a daily spontaneous awake trial (SAT) combined with daily spontaneous breathing trial (SBT), unless they are on paralytic agents. Indications that patients are ready for SBT:

- Minimal ventilator settings (PEEP ≤8 and FiO2 <50%).
- Shock state improving/resolving.
- Cardiac ischemia and/or pulmonary edema have resolved.
- Patients with acute brain injuries must have intracranial pressures controlled.
- Therapeutic hypothermia process completed.
- CXR improving.

Stop SBT if (any of the following are met):

- Develops tachycardia requiring any management or >140 bpm.
- Tachypnea >35 or consider increasing pressure support ventilation (PSV).
- Development of arrhythmia.
- Increasing vasopressor requirements.

Consider extubation when the reason(s) the patient was intubated is reversed or significantly improved and when all of the following are met:

- The patient is awake and able to follow commands. (Neurologically impaired patients can be challenging to assess for extubation. Seek expert consultation.)
- Minimal secretions.
- Patient can lift head off the bed and has a strong cough.
- Rapid shallow breathing index (RSBI) = TV/RR <105. (RSBI <105 on SBT can be expected to be successful approximately 78% of the time.)
- Although less predictive of successful extubation, some clinicians still like to know the following parameters:
  - Negative inspiratory force (NIF) > −20 cmH2O – measurement of respiratory muscle strength (the more negative the number, the stronger the patient's muscles)
  - Vital capacity > 10 mL/kg
  - ETT cuff leak present

ASTHMA

Asthma exacerbations may require an emergency department visit and possible admission when peak expiratory flow (PEF) is 40% to 69% of predicted. Hospital and/or ICU admission is likely when PEF is <40% of predicted.

For moderate exacerbation interventions for PEF 40% to 69% or moderate symptoms:

1. Oxygen to keep oxygen saturation >90%.
2. Inhaled SABA via MDI or nebulizers hourly.
3. Start oral corticosteroids .5 to 1 mg/kg/d of prednisone or prednisone equivalents.

For severe exacerbations for PEF <40% or severe symptoms at rest, accessory muscle use, retractions:

1. Oxygen to keep oxygen saturation >90%.
2. Inhaled SABA via MDI or nebulizers Q 20 minutes; if remains refractory, may increase to continuous nebulizer at 10 to 20 mg/hr till subjectively feeling better.
3. Start IV or oral corticosteroids .5 to 1 mg/kg/d of prednisone or prednisone equivalents.
4. Ipratropium MDI or nebulizer Q 20 minutes or continuously.
5. For patients failing to improve with maximal therapy, consider inhaled Heliox mixture or intravenous magnesium as adjunctive therapies, although data to support is limited.
6. Intubate if the PaCO2 normalizes or if the patient becomes hypercarbic or somnolent.

Upper respiratory tract infections (URI)—including viral illnesses—decreased compliance with medications, exposures to inhalants such as smoke, woodstoves, vaping, and so forth are known common triggers. Prior to discharge, engage the patient and/or family to identify which trigger precipitated the asthma exacerbation to prevent recurrence. Be sure to discuss and update an asthma management plan at time of discharge.

Fast Facts

A patient in status asthmaticus should have an elevated respiratory rate such that they develop a respiratory alkalosis on ABG. If a patient normalizes their $PaCO_2$, becomes hypercapneic, or shows signs of hypercapnia such as sleepiness/drowsiness, they require intubation as they are becoming fatigued and will experience respiratory arrest without prompt intervention.

PNEUMONIA

AG-ACNPs will routinely diagnose and manage patients with pneumonia. Differentiating between viral and bacterial pneumonia and other similar diagnoses, such as COPD or heart failure exacerbations, requires repetition with conscious review of clinical findings. Furthermore, the AG-ACNP then needs to be able to differentiate between community-acquired pneumonia (CAP), hospital-acquired pneumonia (HAP), and ventilator-associated pneumonia (VAP), as treatment regimens for CAP differ significantly from HAP and VAP (see Table 9.7).

Table 9.7

Definition of CAP, HAP, VAP		
CAP	**HAP**	**VAP**
Diagnosed within 48 hours of admission.	Diagnosed 48 hours or more after hospitalization or within 48 hours of discharge from the hospital.	Diagnosed 48 hours or more after intubation or within 48 hours after removal from ventilator.

Note: Healthcare-associated pneumonia (HCAP) terminology has been abandoned to focus on risk factors and need for MRSA or pseudomonal coverage. Send MRSA nasal swab and review prior cultures for previous pseudomonas infections and/or antibiotic resistances. Focus on de-escalation of antibiotics if cultures are negative.

CAP, community-acquired pneumonia; HAP, hospital-acquired pneumonia; MRSA, methicillin-resistant *Staphylococcus aureus*; VAP, ventilator-associated pneumonia.

Diagnosis:

Classic signs of pneumonia include fever/chills, cough, increased oxygen requirements, increased sputum production, and an infiltrate on chest x-ray (see Table 9.8). Procalcitonin will be elevated in bacterial pneumonia but not viral pneumonia, unless concurrent bacterial pneumonia is superimposed on viral pneumonia. Procalcitonin should be used to determine when to cease antibiotic administration, not whether or not to initiate antibiotics.

Aspiration of gastric fluids can cause aspiration pneumonitis, an inflammation of the lining of the lungs, but does not initially indicate a pneumonia or require treatment. Aspiration pneumonitis can subsequently progress into pneumonia in approximately 72 hours. Treatment of aspiration pneumonia should then include coverage of anaerobic organisms.

Knowing when to admit a patient to the hospital can be challenging. Use of a scoring system is helpful. The CURB-65 and/or pneumonia severity index (PSI) can help guide clinicians to safe dispositions for their patients (see Exhibits 9.1 and 9.2).

Table 9.8

Severe Community-Acquired Pneumonia Is Defined as 1 Major or 3 Minor Criteria

Major criteria	Minor criteria
• Septic shock with vasopressor requirement • Respiratory failure requiring mechanical ventilation	• Respiratory rate ≥30 breaths/min • PaO2/FiO2 ratio ≤250 • Multilobar infiltrates • Confusion/disorientation • Uremia (blood urea nitrogen level ≥20 mg/dL) • Leukopenia* (white blood cell count <4,000 cells/µL) • Thrombocytopenia (platelet count <100,000/µL) • Hypothermia (core temperature <36 °C) • Hypotension requiring aggressive fluid resuscitation

Exhibit 9.1

CURB-65 Scoring System

Symptom	Points
Confusion	1
Urea (BUN >19 mg/dL)	1
Respiratory rate ≥30	1
SBP <90 mmHg or DBP ≤60	1

(continued)

Exhibit 9.1

CURB-65 Scoring System (*continued*)

Symptom	Points
Age ≥65	1

TOTAL SCORE:

Interpretation:

– score 0–1 = 1.5% mortality—outpatient management

– score 2 = 9.2% mortality—inpatient vs. observation

– score ≥3 = 22% mortality—inpatient admission

– Score 4 or 5—consider ICU admission

BUN, blood urea nitrogen; DBP, diastolic blood pressure; SBP, systolic blood pressure.

Exhibit 9.2

Pneumonia Severity Index

Characteristic	Points
Age	
• Men	Years
• Women	Years – 10
Nursing home resident	+10
Coexisting illness	
• Neoplastic disease	+30
• Liver disease	+20
• Congestive heart failure	+10
• Cerebrovascular disease	+10
• Chronic renal disease	+10
Physical exam findings	
• Acutely altered mental state	+20
• Respiratory rate ≥30/min	+20
• SBP <90 mmHg	+20
• Temperature <35 or ≥40 °C	+15
• Heart rate ≥125	+10
Laboratory and radiographic findings	
• Arterial pH <7.35	+30
• BUN ≥30 mg/dL	+20

(*continued*)

Exhibit 9.2

Pneumonia Severity Index (*continued*)

Characteristic	Points
• Sodium <130 mEq/L	+20
• Glucose >250 mg/dL	+10
• Hemoglobin <9 gm/dL (hematocrit <30%)	+10
• PaO2 <60 or O2 saturation ≤90%	+10
• Pleural effusion on CXR	+10

TOTAL SCORE:

Interpretation:

Score	Risk class	Mortality (%)	Recommended site of care
<50	I	.1	Outpatient
51–70	II	.6	Outpatient
71–90	III	2.8	Outpatient/Observation
91–130	IV	8.2	Inpatient
>130	V	29.2	Inpatient

ACUTE RESPIRATORY DISTRESS SYNDROME

Acute respiratory distress syndrome (ARDS) is a clinical syndrome triggered by either direct or indirect insults to the lung that cause acute inflammation and lead to increased vascular permeability and interstitial edema, resulting in refractory hypoxemia (see Table 9.9). Precipitating factors are listed in Table 9.9. The Berlin definition in Table 9.10 outlines the clinical criteria and severity of illness.

The PaO2 to FiO2 ratio, commonly referred to as the P:F ratio, is used to determine severity of ARDS and clinical treatments.

P:F ratio = arterial PaO2 divided by FiO2 (expressed as a decimal)

Example: ABG 7.35, PaCO2 45, PaO2 60 on 60% FiO2

= PaO2 60/FiO2 .6 = P:F ratio of 100

Early Management of ARDS

- Shift to low tidal volume 4 to 6 mL/kg.
- Higher levels of PEEP.
- Keep plateau pressures <30.
- Wean FiO2 to goal FiO2 <50%, for saturation 88% to 92% (goal may be higher in brain-injured patients).

Table 9.9

Precipitating Factors of ARDS	
Direct	**Indirect**
• Blunt chest trauma	• Sepsis
• Aspiration	• Shock—any type
• Pneumonia	• Transfusion-related ALI
• Drowning	• Pancreatitis
• Toxic inhalation	• Drugs/contrast
• Embolic events	• Head injury
	• Burns
	• Eclampsia
	• Neurogenic
	• High altitude

ARDS, acute respiratory distress syndrome.

Table 9.10

Berlin Definition and Severity of ARDS	
Timing	Within 1 week of a known clinical insult or worsening respiratory symptoms
Chest imaging	Bilateral opacities, not fully explained by effusions, lobar or lung collapse or nodules
Origin of edema	Respiratory failure not fully explained by cardiac failure or fluid overload (need objective assessment; i.e., ECHO to exclude hydrostatic edema if no risk factors present)
Oxygenation	
Mild	PaO_2/FiO_2 <200 or ≤300 mmHg with PEEP or CPAP >5 cm H_2O
Moderate	PaO_2/FiO_2 <100 or ≤200 mmHg with PEEP >5 cm H_2O
Severe	PaO_2/FiO_2 <100 with PEEP >5 cm H_2O

ARDS, Acute respiratory distress syndrome.

- Conservative fluid management (minimize volume in antibiotics, concentrate continuous infusions, eliminate fluids used to keep veins open [KVO]).
- Early prone positioning, 16 hours prone, 8 hours supine.
- Sedate (with daily awakening trials).
- Permissive hypercapnia (tolerate hypercarbia with pH >7.20).
- Refractory hypoxemia or ventilator dyssynchrony may require neuromuscular blockade (no daily awakening trials while paralyzed).
- Consider venous-to-venous extracorporeal membrane oxygenation (V–V ECMO).

Table 9.11

Light's Criteria to Differentiate Between Transudate vs. Exudate

	Transudate	Exudate
Pleural to serum protein ratio	<.5	≥.5
Pleural to serum LDH	<.6	≥.6
Pleural fluid LDH	<2/3 upper limit of normal	≥2/3 upper limit of normal
Main causes	• Heart failure • Hypoalbuminemia • Cirrhosis • Nephrotic syndrome	• Malignancy • Infection • Pneumonia • Tuberculosis • Fungal • Empyema • Pancreatitis • Esophageal rupture • Chylothorax/Hemothorax • Post-CABG

CABG, coronary artery bypass graft; LDH, lactic dehydrogenase.

PLEURAL EFFUSION

Pleural effusions are commonly noted on chest x-rays for a wide variety of patient conditions. Differentiating between transudative and exudative is an essential skill for AG-ACNPs (see Table 9.11). Using Light's criteria can assist clinicians in determining the etiology of the effusion. To calculate this, concurrent testing of serum and pleural fluid for protein, and lactic dehydrogenase (LDH) is required. Use a phone app or online calculator to aid in this process.

Fast Facts

Use Light's criteria to assist in determining the etiology of the pleural effusion.

In summary, management of patients with acutely decompensating respiratory conditions is a fundamental skill every AG-ACNP must possess, not just those NPs who are working in ICUs. Oftentimes ICU beds are a limited resource and may not be readily available for urgent transfer or admission; thus, the hospitalist or specialty service line AG-ACNPs need to manage these patients until a bed becomes available.

References

Chatburn, R. L., El-Khatib, M., & Mireles-Cabodevila, E. (2014). A taxonomy for mechanical ventilation: 10 Fundamental maxims. *Respiratory Care, 59*(11), 1747–1763.

Fine, M. J., Auble, T. E., Yealy, D. M., Hanusa, B. H., Weissfeld, L. A., Singer, D. E., Coley, C. M., Marrie, T. J., & Kapoor, W. N. (1997). A prediction rule to identify low-risk patients with community-acquired pneumonia. *New England Journal of Medicine, 336*(4), 243–250. https://doi.org/10.1056/nejm199701233360402

Metlay, J. P., Waterer, G. W., Long, A. C., Anzueto, A., Brozek, J., Crothers, K., Cooley, L. A., Dean, N. C., Fine, M. J., & Flanders, S. A. (2019). Diagnosis and treatment of adults with community-acquired pneumonia. An official clinical practice guideline of the American Thoracic Society and Infectious Diseases Society of America. *American Journal of Respiratory and Critical Care Medicine, 200*(7), e45–e67.

Kalil, A. C., Metersky, M. L., Klompas, M., Muscedere, J., Sweeney, D. A., Palmer, L. B., Napolitano, L. M., O'Grady, N. P., Bartlett, J. G., Carratalà, J., El Solh, A. A., Ewig, S., Fey, P. D., File, T. M. Jr., Restrepo, M. I., Roberts, J. A., Waterer, G. W., Cruse, P., Knight, S. L., & Brozek, J. L. (2016). Management of adults with hospital-acquired and ventilator-associated pneumonia: 2016 Clinical practice guidelines by the Infectious Diseases Society of America and the American Thoracic Society. *Clinical Infectious Diseases, 63*(5), e61–e111. https://doi.org/10.1093/cid/ciw353

Holguin, F. (2017). Asthma. In S. J. McKean, J. J. Ross, D. D. Dressler, & D. B. Scheurer (Eds.), *Principles and Practice of Hospital Medicine* (2nd ed., pp. 1876–1886). McGraw Hill Education.

Kummerfeldt, C. E., Pastis, N. J., & Huggins, J. T. (2017). Pleural diseases. In S. J. McKean, J. J. Ross, D. D. Dressler, & D. B. Scheurer (Eds.), *Principles and Practice of Hospital Medicine* (2nd ed., pp. 1923–1931). McGraw Hill Education.

Papazian, L., Aubron, C., Brochard, L., Chiche, J. D., Combes, A., Dreyfuss, D., Forel, J. M., Guérin, C., Jaber, S., Mekontso-Dessap, A., Mercat, A., Richard, J. C., Roux, D., Vieillard-Baron, A., & Faure, H. (2019, 13 June 2019). Formal guidelines: Management of acute respiratory distress syndrome. *Annals of Intensive Care, 9*(1), 69. https://doi.org/10.1186/s13613-019-0540-9

Saeed, F. & Lasrado, S. (2021). Extubation. In *StatPearls [Internet]*. StatPearls Publishing. www.ncbi.nlm.nih.gov/books/NBK539804

10

Renal Acute Care

A hospitalized patient's baseline renal function can worsen secondary to acute conditions of dehydration, sepsis, and heart failure. Additionally, diagnostic and therapeutic interventions such as the use of contrast dye to enhance imaging modalities and medications like diuretics, antibiotics, or antihypertensives can propagate renal dysfunction. Acute kidney injury is one of the most common complications experienced by acutely and critically ill patients.

In this chapter, you will learn to

- identify the stages of chronic kidney disease;
- identify pre-, intra-, and postrenal causes of acute kidney injury;
- define the diagnostic criteria for acute kidney injury;
- classify acute kidney injury using RIFLE criteria;
- evaluate patient findings for the indications associated with the need for hemodialysis and continuous renal replacement therapy; and
- differentiate anion-gap and nonanion-gap metabolic acidosis.

CHRONIC KIDNEY DISEASE

Chronic kidney disease (CKD) affects approximately 13% of the population and is associated with significant morbidity, mortality, and cost. Serum creatinine is an unreliable marker of renal function, as normal values vary with gender, age, and muscle mass. Glomerular filtration rate (GFR) is the preferred marker to assess and monitor renal function. CKD is defined as a GFR >60 mL/min or kidney dysfunction including

Table 10.1

Stages of Chronic Kidney Disease		
Stage	Description	GFR (mL/min/1.73 m^2)
1	Kidney damage with normal or increased GFR	≥90
2	Kidney damage with mild decreased GFR	60–89
3	Moderate decrease in GFR	30–59
4	Severe decrease in GFR	15–29
5	Kidney failure	<15 or HD

GFR, glomerular filtration rate.

proteinuria, hematuria, or abnormal imaging with GFR <90 mL/min (see Table 10.1).

COCKCROFT-GAULT FORMULA

GFR is not easily measured, thus the Cockcroft-Gault formula is used to estimate creatinine clearance (CrCl) and provide an approximate renal function in patients with stable CKD. This formula is not designed for use in acute kidney injury. It is found on many apps and online calculators.

The Cockcroft-Gault formula is: CrCl (male) = [(140-age) × weight in kg]/(PCr × 72)

Creatinine clearance (CrCl) is an estimate of GFR; however, CrCl is slightly higher than true GFR because creatinine is secreted by the proximal tubule (in addition to being filtered by the glomerulus). The additional proximal tubule secretion falsely elevates the CrCl estimate of GFR.

Fast Facts

Many medications, particularly antibiotics, are nephrotoxic, requiring renal dosing. Don't be shy about checking with a clinical pharmacist for guidance on dosing.

ACUTE KIDNEY INJURY

Acute kidney injury (AKI) occurs in 25% of critically ill patients due to sepsis, hypotension, and nephrotoxic agents. Nephrotoxic agents include antibiotics, diuretics, antihypertensives, and contrast dye used to enhance radiographic-imaging modalities. Patients of older age (>65 years) are at most risk for AKI.

Prerenal Causes of AKI Include:

- Hypovolemia—from diarrhea, vomiting, hemorrhage, poor oral fluid intake, sepsis, overdiuresis, high insensible losses
- Decreased cardiac output to kidneys: congestive heart failure, renal artery stenosis, aortic dissection
- Decreased renal perfusion due to medications

Intrarenal Causes of AKI Include:

Acute tubular necrosis (ATN)

- ischemia

Toxins

- drugs (vancomycin, aminoglycosides)
- heavy metals

Glomerular disease

- glomerulonephritis
- lupus
- vasculitis

Vascular disease

- atherosclerosis
- aortic aneurysms
- thromboses

Microvascular disease

- embolic disease
- heparin-induced thrombocytopenia
- disseminated intravascular coagulation
- thrombotic thrombocytopenic purpura
- hemolytic uremic syndrome
- HELLP syndrome (hemolysis, elevated liver enzymes, and low platelets)

Macrovascular disease

- renal artery occlusion
- abdominal aortic aneurysm

Interstitial disease

- allergic reaction to drugs
- autoimmune disease

- connective-tissue diseases
- pyelonephritis, infiltrative disease
- lymphoma or leukemia

Postrenal Causes of AKI Include:

- Prostatic hypertrophy (benign or malignant)
- cervical cancer
- obstruction (e.g., renal calculi, urate crystals)
- pelvic mass
- intraluminal bladder mass (e.g., clot, tumor)
- neurogenic bladder
- urethral strictures

Fast Facts

The older population is at an increased risk for AKI due to reduced numbers of functioning nephrons, which is expected during the aging process. Therefore, it is imperative to calculate creatinine clearance in older adults despite normal creatinine levels.

Diagnostic Criteria of AKI:

- Increase of serum creatinine by >.3 mg/dL within 48 hours, OR
- Increase serum creatinine to >1.5× baseline which is known or presumed to have occurred in last 7 days, OR
- Urine output <.5 mL/kg/hr × 6 hours (see Table 10.2).

Table 10.2

RIFLE Classification of AKI	
Risk	Increase in serum creatinine level × 1.5 or decrease in GFR by 25% or urine output (UO) .5 mL/kg/hr for 6 hours
Injury	Increase in serum creatinine level × 2.0 or decrease in GFR by 50% or UO <.5 mL/kg/hr for 12 hours
Failure	Increase in serum creatinine level × 3.0, decrease in GFR by 75%; or serum creatinine level >4 mg/dL with acute increase of .5 mg/dL; UO <.3 mL/kg/hr for 24 hours or anuria for 12 hours
Loss	Persistent AKI, complete loss of kidney function >4 weeks
End-stage kidney disease	Complete loss of kidney function >3 months

AKI, acute kidney injury; GFR, glomerular filtration rate; RIFLE, Risk, Injury, Failure, Loss of kidney function, and End-stage kidney disease.

Table 10.3

	AKIN Classification System for AKI	
Stage	Serum creatinine	Urine output
1	Increased creatinine >.3 mg/dL or increase 150–200% from baseline	<.5 mL/kg/hr for >6 hours
2	Increase 200–300% from baseline	<.5 mL/kg/hr for >12 hours
3	Increase >300% from baseline or creatinine >4.0 mg/dL	>.3 mL/kg/hr for 24 hours or anuria for 12 hours

AKI, acute kidney injury; AKIN, acute kidney injury network.

The acute kidney injury network (AKIN) classification is a modified version of the RIFLE classification, and was designed to increase the sensitivity and specificity of the AKI diagnosis (see Table 10.3).

Contrast-induced nephropathy (CIN) typically occurs about 48 hours after receiving IV contrast. Repeated contrast exposure within a few hours to days of each other can increase the incidence of CIN. Prophylaxis with IV hydration with normal saline before, during, and shortly after contrast administration can reduce the incidence of CIN. Other interventions such as bicarbonate or N-acetylcysteine (mucomyst) are not necessary.

Renal Assessment Commonly Includes:

- Urinalysis
- Urine sodium and creatinine
- Serum sodium and creatinine
- Calculate the fractional excretion of sodium (FeNa) or, if a loop diuretic is given, can calculate fractional excretion of urea (FeUrea) with the following formulas or use an app.
  - $FeNa = (UNa \times PCr)/(UCr \times PNa) \times 100$
    - <1% indicates prerenal cause
    - >1% indicates renal cause
  - $FeUrea = (UBUN \times PCr)/(PBUN \times UCr) \times 100$
    - <20% to 30% indicates prerenal cause
    - >40% to 70% indicates renal cause
- Consider renal ultrasound to rule out hydronephrosis, renal mass, or cysts.

Acute kidney injury can lead to anuria and may result in hyperkalemia, volume overload, or metabolic acidosis, which requires urgent or emergent interventions. Severe hyperkalemia can lead to cardiac arrest. Thus, monitor for peaked T waves and conduction delays that manifest as widening QRS. If left untreated, it will progress into the sine wave and ultimately lead to cardiac arrest and death. AG-ACNPs must be able to immediately recognize and treat severe hyperkalemia (see Tables 10.4 and 10.5). Temporizing agents

Table 10.4

Treatment of Hyperkalemia

Agent and Dose	Mechanism	Onset	Duration
Calcium gluconate 10 mL of 10% solution infused over 2–3 minutes	Stabilize cell membranes	1–3 minutes	30–60 minutes
D50% 50 mL IV and regular insulin 10 units IV	Redistribution	10–20 minutes	4–6 hours peak, 30–60 minutes
Albuterol 10–20 mg nebulized	Redistribution	30 minutes	2–4 hours peak, 90 minutes
Bicarbonate 150 mEq IV	Redistribution	30 minutes	2–3 hours
Kayexalate 15–60 gm PO/PR	Removal	1–2 hours	variable
Patiromer 8.4–25.2 gm PO daily—for chronic hyperkalemia	Removal	7 hours	variable
Sodium zirconium cyclosilicate 10–15 gm/d PO	Removal	1 hour	variable
Dialysis or CRRT	Removal	Immediate	Same as dialysis treatment

CRRT, continuous renal replacement therapy.

Table 10.5

AEIOU Indications for Dialysis

Acidosis	pH <7.2 and/or refractory to bicarbonate
Electrolytes	Hyperkalemia
Ingestions	salicylate, ethylene glycol
Overload	volume overload
Uremia	causing encephalopathy, pericarditis, seizures, platelet dysfunction with severe bleeding, intractable nausea/vomiting

simply redistribute the potassium back into the cells but does not remove it from the body, and hyperkalemia can recur. Thus, be sure to follow temporizing agents with removal agents to remove excess potassium from the body.

Continuous Renal Replacement Therapy (CRRT)

CRRT is preferred in patients who are hemodynamically unstable. CRRT can be either continuous arterial-to-venous hemodialysis (CAVHD) or continuous venous-to-venous hemodialysis (CVVHD). CVVHD is preferred over intermittent hemodialysis. Advantages of CRRT include a lower risk of hemodynamic instability and more control of fluid and metabolic status. Disadvantages are high cost, increased nursing care, restricted patient mobility, and a need for anticoagulation to the filter, circuit, or systemically to prevent the circuit from clotting.

Indications for CRRT:

- Refractory hypervolemia
- Hyperkalemia (K >6.5 mEq/L)
- Acidosis (pH <7.1)
- Azotemia (BUN >100 mg/dL)
- Severe hyper-/hyponatremia (Na >155 mEq/L or <120 mEq/L, respectively)
- Uremia

Fast Facts

Use extreme caution when prescribing electrolyte replacement in any patient with acute kidney injury or oliguria. Potassium replacement can lead to hyperkalemia and arrhythmias, leading to the need for emergent dialysis.

VOLUME STATUS

Determination of volume status can be challenging. How best to assess fluid balance is commonly debated by providers during daily rounds. Several modes of assessment may be required to figure out the intravascular status of fluids. Central venous pressure (CVP) is not a reliable measurement as it can be affected by patient position, acute or chronic cardiovascular disease, and intrathoracic pressures. Daily weights are also not reliable due to variations in linens/pillows and bed position. Additionally, daily weight does not specify the location of the volume as intra- or extravascular. Common modes of intravascular volume assessment include:

- Pulse pressure variation
- Inferior vena cava (IVC) variability
- The FloTrac®/Vigileo device uses arterial pressure waveform analysis to calculate stroke volume and cardiac output
- Esophageal Doppler monitor (measures thoracic aortic blood velocity to calculate stroke volume and cardiac output)
- Passive leg raises
- Pulmonary artery catheter

No single measurement device is exact, thus vital signs, physical assessment, chest x-rays, laboratory data, and clinical judgment all need to be considered in conjunction with these measuring devices to determine if the patient is hypovolemic, euvolemic, or hypovolemic.

FREE WATER DEFICIT

Many hospitalized patients can become hypernatremic, which is commonly due to dehydration from poor oral intake or GI losses, renal losses from overdiuresis, central or nephrogenic diabetes insipidus, or post-ATN polyuria. To estimate the volume of water in liters required to correct dehydration-related hypernatremia, use the water-deficit equation:

$$[(Serum\ Na - 140)/140] \times 0.6 \times Body\ Weight\ in\ Kg$$

Free water deficit should be replaced over a few days, with a maximum of half over the first 24 hours to avoid overcorrection. Replacing free water enterally is least costly via PO intake or nasogastric tube. For patients who have a nonfunctioning gastrointestinal tract due to ileus or NPO status, administration of dextrose 5% in water (D5W) continuous infusion should be used. Half normal saline (.45% NS) can also be administered. Avoid administration of free water in acutely brain-injured patients, as free water can lead to additional cerebral edema and herniation syndrome. Monitor daily sodium levels, and wean off free water as the sodium level reaches <145 mg/dL.

ACID/BASE BALANCE

Arterial blood gas (ABG) or venous blood gas (VBG) sampling can be used to assess acid-base status. The pH, $PaCO_2$, HCO_3, and base excess results are used to diagnose respiratory or metabolic acidosis or alkalosis. Additionally, ABGs are the primary tool used to adjust ventilator settings. The following are normal values for ABGs:

- pH = 7.35 to 7.45
- pCO_2 = 35 to 45 mmHg
- pO_2 = 75 to 100 mmHg
- HCO_3^- = 22 to 26 mEq/L
- O_2 saturation = >95%
- Base excess = −2 to +2

AG-ACNPs must have the ability to quickly and efficiently interpret an ABG. Follow these steps:

1. Assess the pH.
2. Determine if the pH is normal, acidotic, or alkalotic.
3. $PaCO_2$ level determines ventilation; a high level means insufficient ventilation, which will lower the pH and vice versa.

4. HCO3- level signifies metabolic/renal effect. A low HCO3- is decreasing the pH and vice versa.
5. If the pH is acidotic, identify the number that corresponds with a lower pH. Metabolic acidosis is depicted with a low HCO3-. In respiratory acidosis, the CO2 will be high. If the patient is compensated, the HCO3- will also be high.
6. If the pH is alkalotic, again, determine which value is causing this. In respiratory alkalosis, the CO2 is low; in metabolic alkalosis, the HCO3- is high. Compensation by either system will be opposite; for respiratory alkalosis, the metabolic response should be a low HCO3- and for metabolic alkalosis, the respiratory response should be a high CO2.
7. If the pH level is normal but the PaCO2 and/or bicarb are not within normal limits, a mixed disorder can exist.

Metabolic Acidosis

Primary metabolic acidosis can be caused by many conditions. There are two types of metabolic acidosis: high anion-gap acidosis and nonanion-gap acidosis.

The formula to calculate an anion gap: $[Na]-([Cl]+[HCO3])$

The presence of an anion gap signifies that there are other anions causing the acidosis. Exploration for the cause of the acidosis is important in order to correctly diagnose and treat the acidosis. Use of the mnemonics MUDPILES and HARD UPS can help the AG-ACNP recall the causes of high anion-gap acidosis and nonanion-gap acidosis, respectively (see Table 10.6).

In summary, hospitalized patients commonly experience renal dysfunction. Acute kidney injury occurs commonly from changes in volume status, hypotension and shock states, contrast and/or other nephrotoxic medications. The kidney maintains acid/base and volume homeostasis.

Table 10.6

Mnemonic for Acidosis	
High anion-gap acidosis (MUDPILES)	Nonanion-gap acidosis (HARD UPS)
M = Methanol	H = Hyperalimentation (parenteral nutrition)
U = Uremia	
D = DKA	A = Acetazolamide
P = Propylene glycol, paraldehyde	R = Renal tubular acidosis
I = Infection	D = Diarrhea
L = Lactic acidosis	U = Ureteroenteric fistula
E = Ethylene glycol	P = Pancreaticoduodenal fistula
S = Salicylates	S = Spironolactone

It is a fragile organ that warrants AG-ACNPs to pay special attention to prevent or reverse dysfunction.

References

Farkas, J. (2016). *Hypernatremia & dehydration in the ICU*. www.emcrit.org/ibcc/hypernatremia

Hopkins, E., Sanvictores, T., & Sharma S. (2021, 14 September 2020). *Physiology, Acid Base Balance*. StatPearls Publishing. www.ncbi.nlm.nih.gov/books/NBK507807

Huber, W., Schneider, J., Lahmer, T., Küchle, C., Jungwirth, B., Schmid, R. M., & Schmid, S. (2018). Validation of RIFLE, AKIN, and a modified AKIN definition ("backward classification") of acute kidney injury in a general ICU: Analysis of a 1-year period. *Medicine*, *97*(38), e12465–e12465. https://doi.org/10.1097/MD.0000000000012465

Khwaja, A. (2012). KDIGO clinical practice guidelines for acute kidney injury. *Nephron Clinical Practice*, *120*(4), c179–c184. https://doi.org/10.1159/000339789

Lam, A. Q., & Seifter, J. L. (2017). Assessment and management of patients with renal disease. In S. J. McKean, J. J. Ross, D. D. Dressler, D. B. Scheurer (Eds.), *Principles and Practice of Hospital Medicine* (2nd ed., pp. 397–411). McGraw Hill Education.

Lopes, J. A., & Jorge, S. (2013). The RIFLE and AKIN classifications for acute kidney injury: A critical and comprehensive review. *Clinical Kidney Journal*, *6*(1), 8–14. https://doi.org/10.1093/ckj/sfs160

11

Gastrointestinal Acute Care

For most AG-ACNPS, the gastrointestinal (GI) system is a straight-forward and logical system once anatomy and functionality are mastered. This chapter covers common situations such as GI pro-phylaxis indication and gastrointestinal bleeding. Additionally, some of the more challenging aspects of the GI tract are included, such as liver function test interpretation, hepatitis testing inter-pretation, calculating MELD scores, and Ranson's criteria for pancreatitis.

In this chapter, you will learn

- to evaluate patients for the indications to prescribe stress ulcer prophylaxis,
- *Heliobacter pylori (H. pylori)* treatment options,
- to interpret liver function tests,
- to interpret hepatitis laboratory testing, and
- how to calculate a MELD score.

STRESS ULCER PROPHYLAXIS

Critically ill patients are at risk for stress ulcers due to decreased perfusion of the mucosa in the stomach. The mucosal barrier becomes compromised and can no longer block the detrimental effects of hydrogen ions and oxygen radicals during critical illness. Additionally, the risk for developing stress ulcers is heightened when the patient is critically ill or injured. However, patients who can tolerate enteral feedings often do not need GI prophylaxis prescribed.

Table 11.1

Differentiating Signs and Symptoms Between Gastric and Duodenal Ulcers

Gastric ulcers	Duodenal ulcers
• Pain in LUQ and epigastric areas	• Pain in RUQ
• Pain immediately after meals	• Pain 1–2 hours after meals
• Pain does not radiate	• Pain may radiate to back
• Food aggravates pain	• Food may relieve pain
• Weight loss due to reduced intake	• Weight gain may occur
• Hematemesis common	• Hematemesis not common
	• Manifests as melena

LUQ, left upper quadrant; RUQ, right upper quadrant.

Indications for stress ulcer prophylaxis:

- Mechanical ventilation greater than 48 hours
- Glucocorticoid therapy
- History of or current GI bleeding or ulcerations
- Traumatic brain injury
- Spinal cord injury
- Burn injury
- Coagulopathy (INR >1.5, PTT >2× control with platelet count <50,000

Fast Facts

Not all acutely or critically ill hospitalized or anticoagulated patients require GI prophylaxis. Choose wisely, as complications are increasingly being seen with proton pump inhibitors, specifically *clostridium difficile* infections.

GASTROINTESTINAL BLEEDING

Common causes of upper GI bleeding include gastric or duodenal ulcers, esophageal varices, and Mallory-Weiss tears (see Table 11.1). NSAID use, alcohol use/abuse, stress, tobacco use, and caffeine and nicotine use are all commonly associated with upper GI bleeding and need to be explored in the history of present illness (HPI).

Fast Facts

Clinicians can be misled to believe melena is caused by bleeding in the lower GI tract. However, a frequent cause of melanotic stools is brisk upper GI bleeding.

Gastric ulcers are commonly caused by the bacterial infection *H. pylori*, a gram-negative, helically shaped, microaerophilic bacterium usually found in the stomach. A fecal antigen, carbon 13 urea breath test, or serum *H. pylori* sample is needed to diagnose *H. pylori*.

H. pylori Treatment Options:

Option 1:

- PPI BID, plus
- Clarithromycin 500 mg orally (PO) twice daily (BID), and
- Amoxicillin 1,000 mg PO BID.
- Treat for 10 to 14 days.

Option 2:

- PPI BID, plus
- Clarithromycin 500 mg PO BID, and
- Metronidazole 500 mg PO BID.
- Treat for 10 to 14 days.

Option 3:

- Ranitidine 150 mg PO BID, plus
- Bismuth subsalicylate 525 mg PO four times daily (QID), plus
- Metronidazole 250 mg PO QID and tetracycline 500 g QID.
- Treat for 10 to 14 days.

Option 4:

- PPI BID for 10 days, plus
- Amoxicillin 1 gm PO BID for 5 days, followed by
- Clarithromycin 500 mg PO BID and tinidazole 500 mg PO BID for 5 more days.

Common causes of lower GI bleeding include hemorrhoids, diverticulosis, and cancers. Be sure to inquire about family history, weight loss, change in bowel movements, and previous episodes of diverticulosis. Additionally, a common cause of what appears to be a lower GI bleed is actually a brisk upper GI bleed.

Treatment

All patients with GI bleeding should have two large bore IVs, an active type and screen in the blood bank with cross-matched blood available for immediate transfusion, and a GI consult. Coagulation studies should be done, and any coagulopathy should be corrected. See Chapter 12 for anticoagulant reversal agents and dosing. GI bleeding may be severe at times and can require a mass transfusion protocol (MTP) to be executed. Communication with the blood bank is key to ensuring they understand the situation so they can meet the patient's needs. Don't hesitate to call them to apprise them of the situation.

PANCREATITIS

Pancreatitis commonly requires hospitalization for pain management and fluid resuscitation. Evaluation of the cause of pancreatitis is crucial to prevent recurrence. Pancreatitis can be acute or chronic in nature. Severe cases of acute pancreatitis can develop into necrotizing pancreatitis.

Causes

- The most common causes of pancreatitis:
    - cholelithiasis
    - alcohol misuse
- Other causes of pancreatitis include:
    - iatrogenic due to surgery or GI procedures such as endoscopic retrograde cholangiopancreatography (ERCP)
    - metabolic and autoimmune disorders
    - hypertriglyceridemia
    - cancers (including intraductal papillary mucinous neoplasia[IPMN])
    - anatomical abnormalities
    - infection, ischemia
    - trauma
    - medications
- Common medications that induce pancreatitis include:
    - Azathioprine and 6-mercaptopurine
    - ACE inhibitors
    - metformin
    - statins
    - aspirin
    - metronidazole
    - tetracyclines
    - valproic acid

Treatment Recommendations:

- Use goal-directed therapy for fluid management/resuscitation.
- Avoid hydroxyethyl starch (HES) fluids.
- In patients with necrotizing acute pancreatitis, avoid the use of prophylactic antibiotics.
- In patients with acute biliary pancreatitis and no cholangitis, avoid the routine use of urgent ERCP.
- Start oral feeding early (within 24 hours) as tolerated, avoid NPO.
- If unable to feed orally, start enteral rather than parenteral nutrition.
- In patients with severe or necrotizing pancreatitis that requires enteral tube feeding, use either nasogastric (NG) or nasojejunal (NJ) route.

Table 11.2

Ranson and Modified Ranson Criteria Comparison

Ranson criteria for alcoholic pancreatitis	Modified Ranson criteria for gallstone pancreatitis
On admission:	On admission:
• Age over 55 years	• Age over 70 years
• WBC count >16,000 cells/cm	• WBC >18,000 cells/cm
• Blood glucose >200 mg/dL	• Blood glucose >220 mg/dL
• Serum AST >250 IU/L	• Serum AST >250 IU/L
• Serum LDH >350 IU/L	• Serum LDH >400 IU/L
At 48 hours:	At 48 hours:
• Serum calcium <8.0 mg/dL	• Serum calcium <8.0 mg/dL
• Hematocrit fall >10%	• Hematocrit fall >10%
• PaO2 less than 60 mmHg	• BUN increased by 2 or more mg/dL despite IV fluid hydration
• BUN increased by 5 mg/dL or more despite intravenous (IV) fluid hydration	• Base deficit >5 mEq/L
• Base deficit >4 mEq/L	• Sequestration of fluids >4 L
• Sequestration of fluids >6 L	

Score interpretation

0 to 2 points: mortality 0% to 3%; 3 to 4 points: mortality 15%; 5 to 6 points: mortality 40%; 7 to 11 points: mortality nearly 100%.

AST, aspartate aminotransferase; BUN, blood urea nitrogen; LDH, lactate dehydrogenase; WBC, white blood cell.

- In patients with acute biliary pancreatitis, consult surgical team to perform cholecystectomy.
- In patients with acute alcoholic pancreatitis:
  1. perform screening,
  2. brief intervention, and
  3. referral to treatment (SBIRT) during admission.

Ranson's Criteria

The Ranson's criteria are used to assess acute pancreatitis severity and risk for mortality (see Table 11.2). The Ranson's criteria include 11 parameters that are used to score alcoholic pancreatitis. The modified Ranson's criteria include 10 parameters and are used to score pancreatitis due to gallstones.

Five parameters are assessed on admission, and the others are assessed 48 hours after admission. Each positive criterion is one point, with a maximum score of 11 points, whereas,the modified criteria have a maximum score of 10 points.

LIVER DYSFUNCTION

Liver dysfunction can be categorized as acute or chronic conditions. Acute liver failure causes include acute viral infections, toxins or drugs (see Table 11.3), pregnancy-related issues, autoimmune hepatitis, malignancy, hepatic ischemia, vascular, or the aftermath of extensive resection. Chronic liver disease can be caused by alcoholic or nonalcoholic fatty liver disease (NAFLD), viral illnesses (e.g., hepatitis, A, B, C, D, and

Table 11.3

Medications That Can Cause Hepatotoxicity

Category	Drug/drug categories
Over-the-counter agents	• Acetaminophen (Tylenol) • Nonsteroidal anti-inflammatory drugs • Niacin
Antibiotics	• Amoxicillin-clavulanate (Augmentin) • Fluoroquinolones • Isoniazid • Macrolides • Nitrofurantoin (Macrodantin, Macrobid) • Tetracyclines • Trimethoprim-sulfamethoxazole (Bactrim)
Antifungals	• Fluconazole (Diflucan) • Voriconazole (Vfend)
Antivirals	• Antiretrovirals for HIV
Anticonvulsants	• Phenytoin (Dilantin) • Carbamazepine (Tegretol) • Valproic acid (Depakene)
Antihypertensives	• Angiotensin-converting enzyme inhibitors (ACEi)
Lipid-lowering agents	• Statins • Niacin
Other	• Allopurinol (Zyloprim) • Amiodarone (Cordarone) • Metformin (Glucophage) • Methyldopa (Aldomet) • Propylthiouracil • Tamoxifen (Soltamox) • Thioglitazones (pioglitazone, rosiglitazone) • Tricyclic antidepressants
Illicit substances	• Cocaine • 3,4-Methylenedioxymethamphetamine (MDMA), also known as ecstasy • Methamphetamines

E), toxic exposures, heart failure, hyperlipidemia, and ductal obstruction. Viral infections that cause liver dysfunction include hepatitis A, B, C, D, and E; herpes simplex; varicella zoster; cytomegalovirus; and Epstein-Barr viruses. Complications of any liver dysfunction can lead to thrombocytopenia, coagulopathy, and bleeding. Untreated chronic liver dysfunction can also lead to cirrhosis or hepatocellular carcinoma (HCC) and end-stage liver disease (ESLD) (see Tables 11.4 and 11.5 for LFT interpretation and associated conditions.)

Fast Facts

Patients with acute liver failure who develop encephalopathy and coagulopathy should have early referral or transfer to a transplant center. Patients with rapidly progressing encephalopathy should be intubated prior to transfer.

LFT INTERPRETATION

Table 11.4

Patterns of Abnormal LFTs

Condition	ALT	AST	ALP	GGT	Bilirubin
Hepatocellular	↑↑	↑↑	± ↑	± ↑	± ↑
Viral	Often AST < ALT		± ↑	± ↑	± ↑
NAFLD	Often AST < ALT		± ↑	± ↑	± ↑
Alcoholic	AST:ALT > 2:1		± ↑	↑	± ↑
Ischemic	↑↑↑	↑↑↑	↑↑	± ↑	↑↑
Cholestatic	± ↑	± ↑	↑↑	↑↑	↑↑

ALP, alkaline phosphatase; ALT, alanine transaminase; AST, aspartate aminotransferase; GGT, Gamma-glutamyl transferase; LFTs, liver function tests; NAFLD, nonalcoholic fatty liver disease.

Table 11.5

Common Liver Tests and Associated Conditions

Liver test:	Commonly elevated in:
AST, ALT	Hepatocellular injury: ethanol, hepatitis, ischemia, NAFLD Acute biliary obstruction

(continued)

Table 11.5

Common Liver Tests and Associated Conditions (*continued*)	
Liver test:	Commonly elevated in:
Alkaline phosphatase (ALP)	Cholestasis, bone disease, pregnancy
Gamma-glutamyl transferase (GGT)	Cholestasis, medications, alcohol
Bilirubin	Acute or chronic liver disease, congenital disorders of bilirubin metabolism

ALT, alanine transaminase; AST, aspartate aminotransferase; NAFLD, Nonalcoholic fatty liver disease.

Table 11.6

Hepatitis B Serology Interpretation	
Laboratory test and result	Interpretation
HBsAG (−) Anti-HBc (−) Anti-HBs (−)	Susceptible to infection
HBsAG (−) Anti-HBc (+) Anti-HBs (+)	Immune from infection
HBsAG (−) Anti-HBc (−) Anti-HBs (+)	Immune due to vaccine
HBsAG (−) Anti-HBc (−) Anti-HBs (−)	Infected*

*If actively infected, check IgM anti-HBc. If positive = acute infection, if negative = chronic infection.

Table 11.7

Hepatitis C Serology Interpretation		
	Anti-HCV	HCV RNA
Nonreactive	Negative	Negative
Current infection	Positive	Positive
Past infection	Positive	Negative

HEPATITIS

Hepatitis are common chronic viral infections, however they can be acutely diagnosed. Thus, AGACNPs need to be able to interpret hepatitis serology testing and diagnose hepatitis B and C (see Tables 11.6 and 11.7).

END-STAGE LIVER DISEASE (ESLD)

Common causes of cirrhosis that lead to ESLD include:

- alcohol-related liver disease
- chronic hepatitis B, C, or D
- nonalcoholic steatohepatitis (NASH)
- autoimmune hepatitis
- bile duct disorders
- inherited disorders such as cystic fibrosis and alpha-1 antitrypsin deficiency
- hemochromatosis
- Wilson's disease
- drugs or toxins

Complications of ESLD include:

- ascites
- portal venous hypertension, which can lead to esophageal and/or gastric varices
- variceal bleeding, leading to hemorrhagic shock
- portal vein thrombosis
- hepatic encephalopathy
- spontaneous bacterial peritonitis
- hepatorenal syndrome
- hepatopulmonary syndrome
- hepatic hydrothorax

Treatment of variceal bleeding:

- EGD with banding or sclerosing agents
- nadolol to decrease portal venous pressure (once bleeding stops and hemodynamically stable)
- IV PPI bolus and infusion for 24 to 72 hours
- octreotide infusion at 50 mcg/hr for 24 to 72 hours; octreotide inhibits release of glucagon, a splanchnic vasodilator
- transjugular intrahepatic portosystemic shunt (TIPS) procedure
- placement of Sengstaken-Blakemore tube (temporizing intervention, with high risk of perforating the esophagus if placed incorrectly)

Diagnosis and Treatment of Ascites:

- Grading of ascites:
  - Grade 1: Mild: ascites only detectable by ultrasound.
  - Grade 2: Moderate: moderate symmetrical distention of the abdomen.
  - Grade 3: Large: provokes marked abdominal distention.
- Diagnostic paracentesis
  - Neutrophil count and culture of ascitic fluid should be done to assess for SBP. A neutrophil count over 250 cells/μL is diagnostic.

Protein can be done to diagnose those at high risk for SBP, and cytology should be done to differentiate from malignant ascites.

- Therapeutic paracentesis.
- Midodrine 10 mg PO Q before meals and at bedtime or every 8 hours if intubated.
- Octreotide—100 mcg SC or IV every 8 hours or continuous infusion @ 25 to 50 mcg/hr for 3 to 5 days.
- Antimineralocorticoid or an aldosterone antagonist (e.g., spironolactone).
- Moderate sodium restriction (4.9–6.9 gm/d).
- Add furosemide as ascites progress from grade 1 to 2 to 3.
- For grade 3 ascites: add albumin for postparacentesis circulatory dysfunction (PPCD) 25% albumin 50 gm IV Q 8 hours × 72 hours.

Treatment of Hepatic Encephalopathy:

- Lactulose—30–45 mL PO TID to QID; start Q 1 to 2 hours till stooling; goal 2 to 3 stools per day.
- Rifaximin—550 mg PO BID.

Prophylaxis and Treatment of SBP:

- Ceftriaxone 1 gm IV Q 8 hours × 7 days.
- Ciprofloxacin 250 mg PO daily.

MELD and MELD-Na Score

The model for end-stage liver disease (MELD) and MELD-Na scores stratify severity of end-stage liver disease for transplant planning and resource allocation. The MELD-Na score also considers the patient's sodium level.

- MELD score = $3.78 \times \ln[\text{serum bilirubin (mg/dL)}] + 11.2 \times \ln[\text{INR}] + 9.57 \times \ln[\text{serum creatinine (mg/dL)}] + 6.43$
- MELD-Na score = $\text{MELD} + 1.32 \times (137 - \text{Na}) - [0.033 \times \text{MELD} \times (137 - \text{Na})]$
- For practicality and efficiency, use a phone app or online calculator to calculate the score.
- Be sure to document this score in daily progress notes, as the values change as the patient's condition changes.
- Patients with ESLD and elevated MELD scores should be referred to a hepatologist for evaluation and management, and possible workup and listing for liver transplant.

In summary, this chapter reviews the more common acute gastrointestinal conditions combined with some of the harder-to-recall details of the GI system. Remember, not all acutely or critically ill hospitalized patients require GI prophylaxis. Use the hepatitis table to study for AG-ACNP boards.

References

Avila, P. & Grace, N. D. (2017). Cirrhosis and its complications. In S. J. McKean, J. J. Ross, D. D. Dressler, & D. B. Scheurer (Eds.), *Principles and Practice of Hospital Medicine* (2nd ed., pp. 1253–1268). McGraw Hill Education.

Basit, H., Ruan, G. J., & Mukherjee, S. (2020, 27 September 2020). *Ranson Criteria.* Stat Pearls Publishing LLC. www.ncbi.nlm.nih.gov/books/NBK482345

Conti-Bellocchi, M. C., Campagnola, P., & Frulloni, L. (2015, 8 August 2015). *Drug-induced acute pancreatitis.* https://www.pancreapedia.org/reviews/drug-induced-acute-pancreatitis

Crockett, S. D., Wani, S., Gardner, T. B., Falck-Ytter, Y., Barkun, A. N., Crockett, S., Feuerstein, J., Flamm, S., Gellad, Z., & Gerson, L. (2018). American Gastroenterological Association Institute guideline on initial management of acute pancreatitis. *Gastroenterology, 154*(4), 1096–1101.

European Association for the Study of the Liver. (2018). EASL Clinical Practice Guidelines for the management of patients with decompensated cirrhosis. *Journal of Hepatology, 69*(2), 406–460.

Mahesheshwari, R. S., Subramanian, R. M., & Ford, R. M. (2017). Acute liver disease. In S. J. McKean, J. J. Ross, D. D. Dressler, & D. B. Scheurer (Eds.), *Principles and Practice of Hospital Medicine* (2nd ed., pp. 1239–1252). McGraw Hill Education.

Screening, Brief Intervention, and Referral to Treatment (SBIRT). (2017, 15 September 2017). *Substance Abuse and Mental Health Services Administration.* www.samhsa.gov/sbirt

12

Hematology/Oncology Acute Care

Many hospitalized patients have hematologic and/or oncologic problems. Anemia is the most common hematologic problem and condition found in acutely and critically ill patients. Hospitalized patients are also at great risk for coagulation problems. Diagnosing and treating coagulopathies is time sensitive, and rapid interventions lead to improved outcomes. Oncological emergencies are rare but do require acute interventions, and may require ICU level of care.

In this chapter, you will learn

- to differentiate between types of anemia,
- to interpret thromboelastogram (TEG),
- indications for blood product transfusion,
- reversal agents for anticoagulants, and
- to diagnose and treat oncological emergencies.

PROPHYLACTIC ANTICOAGULANTS

Deep vein thrombosis (DVT) prophylaxis should be prescribed for all hospitalized patients. All patients should receive mechanical DVT prophylaxis, either sequential compression devices (SCD) or foot compression devices, unless there is a known medical contraindication (e.g., severe thrombocytopenia could result in extensive bruising and intradermal bleeding). In the event of surgery or trauma to one or both legs, the SCDs can be placed on an arm or arms.

Chemoprophylaxis is contraindicated initially for spine and brain trauma surgery, those with severe thrombocytopenia, tPA administration within 24 hours, or active bleeding. These contraindications for chemoprophylaxis should be clearly documented in the chart, including a plan or noting when chemoprophylaxis can be initiated.

Anti-Xa Monitoring

Anti-Xa monitoring for low molecular weight heparin (LMWH) is frequently performed for select patients, including those who are grossly under- or overweight, especially with a body mass index (BMI) over 40 kg/m^2, or are severe burn victims with >30% total body surface area (TBSA) burned. Anti-Xa peak is drawn 4 hours after the third consecutive dose. Goal anti-Xa levels should be 0.2 to 0.4 international units (IU)/mL. Maintaining in this therapeutic range will prevent under- or overcoagulation with LMWH.

ANEMIA

Anemia is one of the most common hematologic disorders seen in hospitalized patients. Determining the type of anemia is important to provide holistic, comprehensive care and for billing purposes. Anemia in hospitalized patients is commonly multifactorial in nature and can be related to frequent laboratory draws, hemodilution from IV fluids or heart failure, surgery or traumatic injuries, and underlying chronic illness (see Tables 12.1 and 12.2). Suspect acute blood loss in hospitalized patients with worsening anemia that reaches criteria for transfusion.

Table 12.1

Comparison of the Most Common Anemias Seen in Hospitalized Patients						
	RBC size	MCV (82–99)	MCH (27–32)	TIBC	Ferritin (10–291)	B12 (130–700)
Iron deficiency	Microcytic	⇩	⇩	⇧	⇩	Normal
B-12 deficiency	Macrocytic	⇧	Normal ⇧	Normal	⇧	⇩
Anemia of chronic disease	Normocytic	Normal	Normal	Normal ⇩	Normal ⇧	Normal

Folate is normal in all three, whereas RBC and hemoglobin are all decreased.
MCH, mean corpuscular hemoglobin; MCV, mean corpuscular volume; RBC, red blood cells; TIBC, total iron-binding capacity.

Table 12.2

	Serum Iron	Serum Ferritin	Transferrin Iron Saturation Percentage	Total Iron-Binding Capacity (TIBC)	Transferrin	Hemoglobin
Comparison of Anemias						
Iron deficiency anemia	⇩	⇩	⇩	⇧	⇧	⇩
Vitamin B12 anemia	⇧	⇧	⇧	⇩	⇩	⇩
Anemia of chronic disease	⇩	⇧	⇩	⇩	⇩	⇩
Hemachromatosis	⇧	⇧	⇧	⇩	⇩	Normal
Sideroblastic anemia	⇧	⇧	⇧	⇩	⇩	⇩
Thalassemia	⇧	⇧	⇧	⇩	⇩	⇩
Porphyria cutanea tarda	⇧	⇧	⇧	⇩	⇩	Normal

Fast Facts

The Choosing Wisely® campaign recommends avoiding daily laboratory testing. Rather, providers should order testing based on the need for the information. If the information will not help the provider make a new diagnosis or change the management plan, then it shouldn't be ordered.

Transfusion Indications

Acute and chronic blood loss can require transfusion. Conservative transfusion therapy has been shown to improve patient outcomes. Thus, transfusion threshold is almost universally accepted as hemoglobin of 7.0 g/dL in hemodynamically stable patients, with a few exceptions (see Table 12.3).

Active bleeding and acute coronary syndrome with active cardiac ischemia are routine exceptions to this rule. The AG-ACNP should understand the expected outcome after transfusion. Each unit of packed red blood cells (PRBCs) should increase the hemoglobin (Hgb) by 1 gm. Thus, if a patient who has a Hgb of 6.8 receives one unit of PRBCs, one would expect the Hgb to increase to 7.8 g/dL. Failure to reach this expected outcome should lead the AG-ACNP to suspect ongoing blood loss.

Hemolysis can occur with or without transfusion reactions. AG-ACNPs should be able to interpret results of testing for hemolysis. See Table 12.4 for interpretation of hemolysis laboratory testing.

Table 12.3

Common Transfusion Thresholds

Hemoglobin <7.0 g/dL	Hemoglobin <8.0 g/dL
• Not actively bleeding	• Active bleeding
• Hemodynamically stable (HR <100, stable BP off vasopressors)	• ACS
• Difficulty obtaining crossmatch–specific blood due to patient's antibodies	• Active cardiac ischemia
• Active treatment for hematological malignancy	• Hemodynamic instability – tachycardia, hypotension, or on vasopressor therapy

ACS, acute coronary syndrome.

Table 12.4

Hemolysis Workup and Expected Results in Hemolysis

Peripheral smear	Schistocytes present
Serum LDH	elevated
Serum haptoglobin	decreased
Unconjugated or indirect bilirubin	increased
Reticulocyte count	increased

Changes in LDH and serum haptoglobin are the most sensitive.
LDH, lactate dehydrogenase.

Hemorrhagic Shock

Hemorrhagic shock and coagulopathies are common conditions that AG-ACNPs must be prepared to manage. Transfusion of blood components in the correct amounts and ratios will lead to improved patient outcomes. Concurrent, prompt reversal of coagulopathies will promote faster hemodynamic stabilization. Massive transfusion protocols, reversal agents, and interpretation of thromboelastograms are important for AG-ACNPs to know or have at their fingertip (see Figure 12.1).

Fast Facts

During acute hemorrhages, be sure to contact a member of the blood bank team to notify them of the situation. Keeping all team members abreast of the situation is key to ensure available products in a timely fashion. Communication allows them to prioritize tasks and mobilize human and other resources to meet multiple patient needs simultaneously.

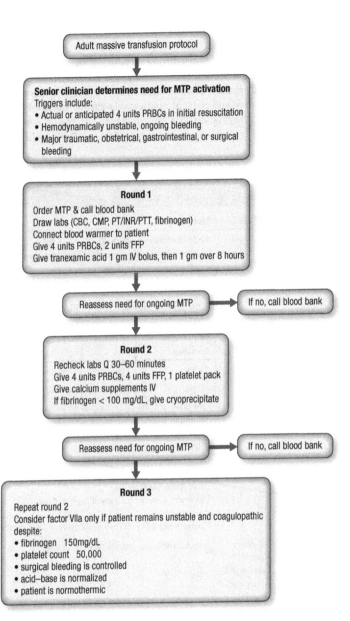

Figure 12.1   Sample massive transfusion protocol

CORRECTION OF COAGULOPATHIES

Achieving hemodynamic stability during an acute hemorrhage requires simultaneous attention to achieving hemostatic control, repletion of blood products and reversal of anticoagulation. During emergent situations, medical history and current medications can be overlooked, as such reversing anticoagulation can be forgotten. For the AG-ACNPs who do not routinely prescribe reversal agents, Table 12.5 will be helpful.

Table 12.5

Reversal Agents for Anticoagulants		
Agent	**Half-life**	**Reversal agent**
Apixaban (Eliquis)	8–15 hours	Andexanet alfa (AndexXa). Indicated if the following criteria are met: • intracranial hemorrhage • last dose of apixaban confirmed within 18 hours • GCS ≥ 7 • no Kcentra, Novoseven, or FEIBA within 48 hours.

Last dose of Apixaban	<8 hours	8–18 hours
≤5 mg	Low dose	Low dose
>5 mg	High dose	Low dose

Low dose: 400 mg IV bolus over 13 minutes, then 480 mg infusion over 2 hours.
High dose: 800 mg IV bolus over 26 minutes, then 960 mg infusion over 2 hours.
Or
4-Factor PCC (KCentra): 25 or 50 units/kg × 1 (maximum 5,000 units).
Use lower dose for patients at high risk for thrombosis.
Contraindicated in HIT within 90 days or active DIC.

Agent	Half-life	Reversal agent
Argatroban	30–50 minutes (prolonged in hepatic impairment)	Stop infusion. No specific reversal agent.
Bivalirudin (Angiomax)	25 minutes (prolonged in renal impairment)	Stop infusion. No specific reversal agent.

(continued)

Table 12.5

Reversal Agents for Anticoagulants (*continued*)

Agent	Half-life	Reversal agent
Dabigatran (Pradaxa)	12–17 hours (prolonged in renal impairment)	Idarucizumab (Praxbind) 5 gm IV × 1 if last dose within 48 hours. If bleeding continues, an additional 5 gm dose may be considered.
Dalteparin (Fragmin)	3–5 hours (prolonged in renal impairment)	Protamine 1 mg per 100 units. Max 50 mg single dose. Consider use of protamine up to 24 hours after dalteparin if renal impairment is present. May consider repeat dosing of .5 mg protamine per 100 units if bleeding continues or aPTT/anti-Xa elevated. Protamine reverses approximately 60–80% of LMWH
Enoxaparin (Lovenox)	4.5–7 hours (prolonged in renal impairment)	Protamine 	Last dose	Dose of protamine	 	<8 hours	1 mg protamine per 1 mg enoxaparin	 	8–12 hours	.5 mg protamine per 1 mg enoxaparin	 Consider use of protamine up to 24 hours after enoxaparin if renal impairment is present. May consider repeat dosing of .5 mg protamine per 1 mg enoxaparin if bleeding continues or aPTT/Anti-Xa remains elevated. Protamine reverses approximately 60–80% of LMWH.
Edoxaban (Savaysa)	10–14 hours (prolonged in renal impairment)	4-Factor PCC (KCentra) 25 or 50 units/kg (max 5,000 units). Indicated if last dose within 72 hours. Use lower dose for patients at high risk of thrombosis.
Fondaparinux (Arixtra)	17–21 hours (prolonged in renal impairment)	No specific reversal agent.

(*continued*)

Table 12.5

Reversal Agents for Anticoagulants (*continued*)

Agent	Half-life	Reversal agent
Heparin (unfractionated intravenous)	1–2 hours	Protamine

Time since last dose	Dose
<30 minutes	1 mg per 100 units heparin
30–120 minutes	0.75 mg per 100 units heparin
>120 minutes	0.375 mg per 100 units heparin

Max dose: 50 mg single dose.
If aPTT remains elevated, consider repeating half initial dose of protamine. When heparin given as an infusion, only the amount of heparin given in the last 2–3 hours should be considered when dosing protamine. If >3 hours since heparin was administered, only consider reversal with protamine if aPTT remains prolonged.
Above does not apply to prophylactic subcutaneous heparin.

Agent	Half-life	Reversal agent
Rivaroxaban (Xarelto)	5–9 hours (prolonged in renal impairment)	Andexanet alfa (AndexXa). Indicated if the following criteria are met: • intracranial hemorrhage • last dose of apixaban confirmed within 18 hours • GCS ≥7 • no Kcentra, Novoseven, or FEIBA within 48 hours

Last dose of Apixaban	<8 hours	8–18 hours
≤10 mg	Low dose	Low dose
>10 mg	High dose	Low dose

Low dose: 400 mg IV bolus over 13 minutes, then 480 mg infusion over 2 hours.
High dose: 800 mg IV bolus over 26 minutes, then 960 mg infusion over 2 hours.
Or
4-Factor PCC (KCentra): 25 or 50 units/kg × 1 (maximum 5,000 units).
Use lower dose for patients at high risk for thrombosis.
Contraindicated in HIT within 90 days or active DIC.

(continued)

Table 12.5

Reversal Agents for Anticoagulants (*continued*)

Agent	Half-life	Reversal agent
Warfarin (Coumadin)	42–72 hours	Vitamin K 10 mg IV × 1 plus one of the following: 4-Factor PCC (Kcentra)

Pretreatment INR	2–3.9	4–6	>6
Kcentra dose (units of Factor IX per kg ABW)	25	35	50
Maximum dose in units:	2,500	3,500	5,000

Kcentra contraindicated in HIT within 90 days or active DIC.
If Kcentra unavailable, may use FFP 10–20 mL/kg or FactorVIIa 2 mg IV × 1.

ABW, actual body weight; aPTT, activated partial thromboplastin time; DIC, disseminated intravascular coagulation; FFP, fresh frozen plasma; GCX, Glasgow Coma Score; HIT, heparin-induced thrombocytopenia; LMWH, low molecular weight heparin; PCC, prothrombin complex concentrate.

Thromboelastogram Interpretation

Thromboelastogram (TEG) is a viscoelastic hemostatic assay that measures the global viscoelastic properties of whole blood from clot formation under low shear stress. It shows interaction of platelets, including aggregation, clot strengthening, fibrin cross-linking, and fibrinolysis (see Table 12.6). It does not correlate with international normalized ratio (INR), activated partial thromboplastin time (aPTTs), or platelet counts. This test can be useful in trauma patients, obstetrics, and early detection of dilutional coagulopathy.

HYPERCOAGULABLE STATES

Disseminated Intravascular Coagulation

Disseminated intravascular coagulation (DIC) is a condition where the patient's own clotting factors are consumed into intravascular clotting, often resulting in thrombocytopenia and uncontrolled bleeding due to decreased available clotting factors. It is also sometimes referred to as

Table 12.6

TEG Interpretation and Treatments

Parameter	Definition	Normal	Problem with:	Treatment
Reaction time (R) value	Time to start clot formation	5–10 minutes	Coagulation factors	FFP
Kinetics (K)	Time for clot to reach fixed strength	1–3 minutes	Fibrinogen	Cryoprecipitate
Alpha or angle	Speed of fibrin buildup	53–72 degrees	Fibrinogen	Cryoprecipitate
Maximum amplitude (MA)	Highest vertical amplitude of the TEG	50–70 mm	Platelets	Platelets (consider DDAVP)
Lysis at 30 minutes (LY30)	Percentage decrease in amplitude at 30 minutes post-MA and measures degree of fibrinolysis	0–8%	Excess fibrinolysis	TXA and/or aminocaproic acid

R, reaction time(s) is the time of latency from start of test to initial fibrin formation; K, kinetics is the time taken to achieve a certain level of clot strength; Alpha, Angle (slope of line between R and K) measures the speed at which fibrin build up and cross-linking takes place; MA, maximum amplitude, represents the ultimate strength of the fibrin clot i.e. overall stability of the clot; LY30, amplitude at 30 minutes is the percentage decrease in amplitude at 30 minutes post-MA r, the fibrinolysis phase.

consumptive coagulopathy. DIC occurs secondary to underlying conditions, which can include:

- trauma, including multitrauma, severe traumatic brain injuries, and burns
- shock states
- sepsis/septic shock
- malignancy, including adenocarcinomas, acute lymphoblastic leukemia, acute promyelocytic leukemia, and acute monocytic leukemia
- severe hemolysis
- placental abruption or retained products of conception, amniotic fluid embolism.

While bleeding may be the most evident sign, organ failure is primarily due to thrombosis of small to midsize vessels. Diagnostic testing for DIC includes:

- PT/INR, aPTT
- D-dimer
- Fibrinogen

- Fibrinogen degradation products
- Platelet count
- Blood cultures as infection is a common trigger of DIC

The treatment of DIC is treatment of the underlying problem. Additionally, patients in DIC will frequently require replacement blood products, including PRBC, PLT, and cryoprecipitate. Serial q8–q12-hour lab testing including CBC and fibrinogen is recommended while the patient remains in DIC.

Fast Facts

Disseminated intravascular coagulation is always secondary to an underlying condition that activates the coagulation cascade. DIC is frequently recognized by overt signs of bleeding; however, the primary pathology of organ failure is due to thrombosis.

Heparin-Induced Thrombocytopenia

Heparin-induced thrombocytopenia (HIT) is most common in surgical or trauma patients with greater than 5-days' use of heparin, whereas HIT causes an antibody reaction. A small percentage of patients will also develop venous or arterial thromboembolism (VTE). When VTEs occur, they can result in loss of digits or limbs, necrosis of skin at injection sites, or adrenal necrosis or anaphylactic reactions. Diagnosis should be based on a pretest probability with the 4T model followed by HIT antibody testing when indicated (see Table 12.7).

Consider testing for HIT antibodies for intermediate or high pretest probability, when platelet counts drop by >50%, or if a thrombotic event is observed within 2 weeks from heparin initiation. Additionally, if HIT is suspected, stop all heparin products and change to nonheparin anticoagulation such as lepirudin, argatroban, danaparoid, bivalirudin, or fondaparinux.

Fast Facts

For patients with heparin-induced thrombocytopenia, consult your clinical pharmacist for dosing on nonheparin anticoagulation.

ONCOLOGIC EMERGENCIES

Many patients are hospitalized for oncologic reasons or are diagnosed with cancer that is incidentally found during diagnostic testing for other

Table 12.7

4T Model to Diagnose Heparin-Induced Thrombocytopenia

4T's	Points
Thrombocytopenia	• 2 – platelet count fall ≥50% and platelet nadir >20 × 10⁹/L • 1 – platelet count fall 30–50% and platelet nadir >10 × 10⁹/L • 0 – platelet count fall <300% and platelet nadir <10 × 10⁹/L
Timing (of platelet decrease)	• 2 – Clear onset between 5–10 days or platelet fall ≤1 day (prior heparin exposure within 30 days) • 1 – Consistent with fall days 5–10 but not clear; onset after 10 days, or fall ≤1 day (prior heparin exposure 30–100 days ago) • 0 – Platelet count fall <4 days without recent exposure
Thrombosis	• 2 – New thrombosis (confirmed); skin necrosis; acute systemic reaction after intravenous unfractionated heparin bolus • 1 – Progressive or recurrent thrombosis; non-necrotizing (erythematous skin lesions; suspected thrombosis [not proven)]) • 0 – None
Other (causes for thrombocytopenia)	• 2 – No apparent cause for thrombocytopenia • 1 – Possible other causes for thrombocytopenia • 0 – Definite other causes for thrombocytopenia

Interpretation: Score 0–3, low pretest probability; 4–5, intermediate pretest probability; 6–8, high pretest probability for HIT.

reasons. Regardless, oncology patients can experience medical emergencies related to their cancers. Table 12.7 outlines the common oncologic emergencies, signs and symptoms, and treatment for each.

Oncologic Conditions, Associated Signs and Symptoms, and Treatment

Metabolic Causes

Tumor Lysis Syndrome

- Associated with hematologic malignancies with high white blood cell counts, particularly acute leukemia and high-grade lymphomas; solid tumors
- Presenting signs and symptoms
  - Azotemia, hyperphosphatemia, hyperkalemia, hyperuricemia, acute renal failure, hypocalcemia
- Treatment
  - Prophylaxis with aggressive IV hydration (>150 mL/hr) and allopurinol
  - Treatment with rasburicase if uric acid >9
  - Treat electrolyte abnormalities

Hypercalcemia

- Associated with multiple myeloma; breast cancer; squamous cell carcinoma of the head or neck, lung, kidney, or cervix
- Presenting signs and symptoms
  - Progressive decline in mental function, weakness, anorexia, thirst, constipation, nausea, vomiting, decreased urine output, possible coma
- Treatment
  - Aggressive IV hydration and loop diuretic
  - IV bisphosphonate with or without calcitonin
  - Refractory cases gallium nitrate or denosumab

Syndrome of inappropriate antidiuretic hormone (SIADH)

- Associated with small cell lung cancer
- Presenting signs and symptoms
  - Hyponatremia, nausea, vomiting, constipation, muscle weakness
- Treatment
  - Fluid restriction
  - Demeclocycline or vasopressin receptor inhibitors (conivaptan or tolvaptan)

Hematologic Causes

Febrile Neutropenia

- Associated with current chemotherapy, some acute leukemias
- Presenting signs and symptoms
  - Axillary/oral temperature ≥100.4 °F (38 °C)
  - an absolute neutrophil count <1,500 cells per mm³ (febrile neutropenia means a fever and neutropenia; mild neutropenia starts at ANC <1.5)
- Treatment
  - Obtain cultures
  - Start broad-spectrum antibiotics
  - Check lactic acid
  - Watch for septic shock; if present, IV fluids 30 mL/kg ABW
  - If hypotensive despite volume, add vasopressors

Hyperviscosity Syndrome

- Associated with Waldenström macroglobulinemia (10–30%), leukemia, multiple myeloma
- Presenting signs and symptoms
  - Spontaneous bleeding, shortness of breath, neurologic deficits (peripheral neuropathies), "sausage-like" hemorrhagic retinal veins, serum viscosity >4 cP (greater than 4 centipoises)
- Treatment
  - Plasmapheresis, hydroxyurea, platelet pheresis, or phlebotomy, depending on etiology

Structural Causes

Superior Vena Cava Syndrome

- Associated with lung cancer, lymphoma, metastatic mediastinal tumors or lymph nodes, indwelling venous catheters
- Presenting signs and symptoms
  - Facial edema, cough, dyspnea at rest, hoarseness, chest and shoulder pain, collateral venous circulation (chest wall)
- Treatment
  - Early: intensive tumor treatment
  - Late: venoplasty, stent

Malignant Epidural Spinal Cord Compression

- Associated with breast cancer, multiple myeloma, lymphoma, lung and prostate cancers
- Presenting signs and symptoms
  - New-onset back pain (worse when lying down)
  - Paraplegia (late presentation)
- Treatment
  - Surgical decompression, chemotherapy

Malignant Pericardial Effusions

- Associated with lung, esophageal, and breast cancers
- Can be seen with lymphoma, leukemia, melanoma, infection, treatment complication, autoimmune reaction
- Presenting signs and symptoms
  - Dyspnea, chest pain, or palpitations
  - Pulsus paradoxus
  - Beck triad (muffled heart sounds, hypotension, increased jugular venous pressure)
- Treatment
  - Pericardiocentesis, pigtail catheter placement or surgical pericardial window.

Treatment Related

Chemotherapy Extravasation

- Associated with current chemotherapy
- Presenting signs and symptoms
  - Pain, erythema, and swelling that progress to blanching, blistering, discoloration, and necrosis of the skin
- Treatment
  - Chemo-specific treatment: Dry cold or warm compresses 20 to 30 minutes once to 4×/day
  - Neutralize with agent-specific antidote

Gastrointestinal Problems

- Associated with current cancer treatment
- Presenting signs and symptoms
  - Abdominal pain, nausea, vomiting, diarrhea, constipation, and dehydration; obstruction; bleeding; weight loss; dehydration
- Treatment
  - Specific symptom management
    - Systemic and topical analgesics, anticholinergics, IVF, antispasmodics, diet, antidiarrheals

Radiation Therapy

- Associated with current radiation therapy (external, temporary internal, permanent internal, or systemic)
- Presenting signs and symptoms
  - Dermatitis, cardiovascular disease, esophagitis, cystitis, sexual dysfunction, depression
- Treatment
  - Specific symptom management
    - Hydrating ointments, topical steroids, cranberry juice, urinary alkalizers

Cytokine Release Syndrome (CRS)

- Associated with CAR-T cell therapy; haploidentical hematopoietic stem cell transplant; therapeutic antibodies (e.g., blinatumomab, obinutuzumab, rituximab, alemtuzumab)
- Noted in association with severe viral infections, including COVID-19
- Presenting signs and symptoms
  - Grade 1—Fever ≥38.0 °C only. May have malaise, myalgias, or arthralgias, but severity not part of grading
  - Grade 2—Temperature ≥38°C plus hypotension that does not require vasopressors and/or hypoxia that requires low-flow nasal cannula (≤6 L/min or blow-by oxygenation)
  - Grade 3—Temperature ≥38 °C plus hypotension that requires one vasopressor (with or without vasopressin) and/or hypoxia requiring high-flow nasal cannula (≥6 L/min), facemask, nonrebreather mask, or Venturi mask that is not attributable to any other cause
  - Grade 4—Temperature ≥38 °C plus hypotension that requires multiple vasopressors (excluding vasopressin) and/or hypoxia requiring positive pressure (e.g., continuous positive airway pressure [CPAP], bilevel positive airway pressure [BiPAP], intubation, and mechanical ventilation)

- Treatment
  - Tocilizumab for grade 2+ and/or glucocorticoids (most common treatment is dexamethasone or Solu-Medrol)

Immune Effector Cell-Associated Neurotoxicity Syndrome (ICANS)

- Occurs in 20% to 70% of all patients treated with CAR-T therapy; occurs in 65% of patients treated with blinatumomab
- CAR-T–related ICANS commonly follows CRS
- Severe ICANS often overlaps with severe CRS
- Presenting signs and symptoms
  - ICANS ranges from mild alterations in the level of consciousness to varying degrees of neurologic dysfunction:
  - Encephalopathy with confusion and behavioral changes
  - Visual and auditory hallucinations
  - Language dysfunction, speech alterations, and apraxia
  - Headache, fatigue, and tremors
  - Dysgraphia and other fine motor impairment
  - Clinical or subclinical seizures, including status epilepticus
  - Cerebral edema with coma
  - Death secondary to malignant cerebral edema
- Treatment
  - Hydrocortisone 100 mg q8h
  - Dexamethasone 10 mg IV up to 4× daily
  - Methylprednisolone 1 mg/kg/d
  - Should be tapered off over 2 to 5 days

Fast Facts

Rapid identification, diagnosis, and treatment of oncologic emergencies is essential to prevent end organ damage.

In summary, AG-ACNPs need to be able to diagnose a variety of anemias, manage hemorrhagic shock, correct coagulopathies, and diagnose and treat a variety of oncologic emergencies. Unless the NP routinely manages these specific conditions, critical information may be difficult to recall during emergent situations. This chapter provides key details to quickly respond to these rapidly evolving situations.

References

Abdelfattah, K., & Cripps, M. W. (2016, 1 September 2016). Thromboelastography and Rotational Thromboelastometry use in trauma. *International Journal of Surgery, 33*, 196–201. https://doi.org/https://doi.org/10.1016/j.ijsu.2015.09.036

De Ruysscher, D., Niedermann, G., Burnet, N. G., Siva, S., Lee, A. W., & Hegi-Johnson, F. (2019). Radiotherapy toxicity. *Nature Reviews Disease Primers*, 5(1), 1–20.

Fredericks, C., Kubasiak, J. C., Mentzer, C. J., & Yon, J. R. (2017). Massive transfusion: An update for the anesthesiologist. *World Journal of Anesthesiology*, 6(1), 14–21.

Levi, M. & Scully, M. (2018). How I treat disseminated intravascular coagulation. *Blood*, 131(8), 845–854. https://doi.org/10.1182/blood-2017-10-804096

Lo, G., Juhl, D., Warkentin, T., Sigouin, C., Eichler, P., & Greinacher, A. (2006). Evaluation of pretest clinical score (4 T's) for the diagnosis of heparin-induced thrombocytopenia in two clinical settings. *Journal of Thrombosis and Haemostasis*, 4(4), 759–765.

Schulman, S., & Meijer, K. (2017). Hypercoagulable states. In S. J. McKean, J. J. Ross, D. D. Dressler, & D. B. Scheurer (Eds.), *Principles and Practice of Hospital Medicine* (2nd ed., pp. 1399–1404). McGraw Hill Education.

Verhovsek, M., & McFarlane, A. (2017). Abnormalities in red blood cells. In S. J. McKean, J. J. Ross, D. D. Dressler, D. B. Scheurer (Eds.), *Principles and Practice of Hospital Medicine* (pp. 1353–1372). McGraw Hill Education.

Warkentin, T. E. (2017). Quantitative abnormalities of platelets: Thrombocytopenia and thrombocytosis. In S. J. McKean, J. J. Ross, D. D. Dressler, & D. B. Scheurer (Eds.), *Principles and Practice of Hospital Medicine* (2nd ed., pp. 1381–1391). McGraw Hill Education.

13

Infectious Disease Acute Care

Infectious disease management of hospitalized patients is a constant challenge for AG-ACNPs to master. Mastery takes years to achieve and requires AG-ACNPs to remain abreast of emerging threats, evolving organisms which create new drug resistances, and new antibiotics being developed. The first step is to learn the normal flora found in each body system, as these commonly become pathogenic. The second step is to learn the clinical practice guidelines for common infections. As you gain experience, you'll add to this knowledge base.

In this chapter, you will learn

- common infectious organisms by body location,
- antibiotic choices prescribed to treat common organisms,
- treatment of common community-acquired infections,
- treatment of common hospital-acquired infections,
- risk factors for fungal infections, and
- to recognize concerning multidrug-resistant organisms.

ORGANISMS

AG-ACNPs will manage viral and bacterial infections as well as possible fungal and protozoal infections. AG-ACNPs will routinely need to differentiate between viral and bacterial infections. Both have similar features of fever, tachycardia, malaise, and can be difficult to distinguish from one another. Assessment for leukocytosis and bandemia, lymphophenia and elevated procalcitonin can aid provider in this process.

Additionally, viral illness can be a nidus to develop bacterial infections such as pneumonia. AG-ACNPs should know body systems, which organisms are normal flora, and which can become pathogenic, causing infections (see Tables 13.1 and 13.2). This is a key concept to being able to empirically treat infections. Common hospital organisms and their associated antibiotic coverage are noted in Tables 13.3 and 13.4.

Table 13.1

Normal Microbiota by System

Location	Community

Skin	– Coagulase-negative staphylococci
	– *Staphylococcus aureus*
	  • Methicillin-sensitive Staphylococcus aureus (MSSA)
	  • Methicillin-resistant Staphylococcus aureus (MRSA)
	– *Streptococcus* spp.
	– *Bacillus* spp.
	– *Candida* spp.
	– Coryneform bacteria
	– *Cutibacterium* spp.

Eyes	– Coagulase-negative staphylococcus – *Staphylococcus aureus* – *Streptococcus* spp. – *Haemophilus* spp.
Ear	– Coagulase-negative staphylococcus – Diphtheroids – *Pseudomonas* spp. – *Enterobacteriaceae*

Nose and upper respiratory tract	– *Staphylococcus* spp.
	  • Coagulase-negative staphylococcus
	  • Staphylococcus aureus
	– *Streptococcus* spp.
	  • Streptococcus viridans
	  • Streptococcus pneumoniae
	– *Haemophilus* spp.
	– *Neisseria* spp.

Mouth and oropharynx	– Anaerobes
	– *Staphylococcus* spp.
	  • Coagulase-negative staphylococcus
	  • Staphylococcus aureus
	– *Streptococcus* spp.
	  • Streptococcus viridans
	  • Streptococcus pneumoniae
	  • Beta-hemolytic streptococci (not group A)
	– *Haemophilus* spp.
	– Diphtheroids

(continued)

Table 13.1

Normal Microbiota by System (*continued*)

Location	Community
	– *Fusobacterium* spp.
	– *Treponema* spp.
	– *Neisseria* spp.
	– *Actinomyces* spp.
Stomach	– *Staphylococcus* spp.
	– *Streptococcus* spp.
	– *Lactobacillus*
	– *Peptostreptococcus*
	– *Candida*
Small bowel	– *Enterococcus*
	– *Enterobacteriaceae*
	– *Lactobacillus* spp.
	– *Bacteroides* spp.
	– *Clostridium* spp.
	– Anaerobes
	– *Candida* spp.
Colon	– *Bacteroides* spp.
	– *Fusobacterium* spp.
	– *Clostridium* spp.
	– *Peptostreptococcus* spp.
	– *Escherichia coli*
	– *Klebsiella* spp.
	– *Proteus* spp.
	– *Lactobacillus* spp.
	– *Enterococcus*
	– *Streptococcus*
	– *Pseudomonas* spp.
	– *Acinetobacter* spp.
	– Coagulase-negative staphylococcus
	– *Staphylococcus aureus*
	– *Actinomyces* spp.
Genitourinary system	– *Lactobacillus* spp.
	– *Streptococcus* spp.
	– *Peptostreptococcus* spp.
	– Diphtheroids
	– *Streptococcus*
	– *Clostridium* spp.
	– *Bacteroides* spp.
	– *Candida* spp.
	– *Gardnerella vaginalis*

Table 13.2

Common Bacterial Infective Organisms by Body Location

Brain–bacterial meningitis	– *Streptococcus pneumoniae* – *Neisseria meningitidis* – *Haemophilus influenzae* – *Streptococcus agalactiae* – *Listeria monocytogenes*
Ear–otitis media	– *Streptococcus pneumoniae*
Eye	– *Staphylococcus aureus* – *Neisseria gonorrhea* – *Chlamydia trachomatis*
Sinus	– *Streptococcus pneumoniae* – *Haemophilus influenza*
Upper respiratory tract	– *Streptococcus pneumoniae* – *Haemophilus influenza*
Pneumonia–community acquired	– *Streptococcus pneumoniae* – *Haemophilus influenza* – *Staphylococcus aureus*
Pneumonia–atypical	– *Mycoplasma pneumoniae* – *Chlamydia pneumoniae* – *Legionella pneumoniae*
Gastritis/ulcers	– *Helicobacter pylori*
Food poisoning	– *Campylobacter jejunum* – Salmonella – Shigella – *Clostridium* – *Staphylococcus aureus* – *Escherichia coli* – *Bacillus cereus*
Skin infections	– *Staphylococcus aureus* – *Streptococcus pyogenes* – *Pseudomonas aeruginosa*
Sexually transmitted diseases	– *Chlamydia trachomatis* – *Neisseria gonorrhea* – *Treponema pallidum*
Urinary tract infections	– *Escherichia coli* – Other *enterobacteriacea* – *Pseudomonas aeruginosa*

ANTIBIOTIC PRESCRIBING TIPS

■ AG-ACNPs are exquisitely positioned to be a primary driver of antibiotic stewardship.

- Use clinical practice guidelines to guide antibiotic prescribing.
- Use antibiograms and local resistance patterns to determine antibiotic selection.
- Keep duration of antibiotics to a minimum necessary to treat the infection.
- Assess culture results and sensitivities daily to de-escalate antibiotics as soon as possible.

Antibiogram

An antibiogram is commonly presented as a table representing antimicrobial susceptibility of a specific microorganism to a battery of antibiotics (see Exhibit 13.1). Every hospital should have this based on the organisms and susceptibility for all the culture results for the institution. Institutions commonly break this information down by inpatient and outpatient, as well as by ICU, floor, and/or emergency department.

Fast Facts

Many antibiotics are cleared through the kidneys, thus special attention to changing renal function is critical to prevent acute kidney injury (AKI) and adequate coverage when AKI is resolving. New NPs should consult with a clinical pharmacist to ensure appropriate antibiotic dosing.

TREATMENT OF COMMON INFECTIONS

Currently five adult guidelines are being revised by the Infectious Diseases Society of America (IDSA), including antimicrobial prophylaxis in surgery, uncomplicated cystitis and pyelonephritis, catheter-associated urinary tract infections, intraabdominal infections, and IV catheters. These guidelines range from 9 to 11 years old and are classified as "archived" and are not included in this resource. *Staphylococcus aureus* bacteremia will be a new resource and is currently in the development phase.

Antimicrobial prophylaxis in surgery—watch for new guidelines emerging from the IDSA.

Clostridioides (Formerly Clostridium) Difficile

Clostridioides difficile infection (CDI) should be suspected when patients have ≥3 new, unformed stools in 24 hours, without other explanations. Stool toxin testing should be part of the diagnostic testing. The first step

Exhibit 13.1

Sample Antibiogram

Gram-Positives January–December 2019

% Susceptible (A blank box can mean that drug is inappropriate for that bacteria or that a simpler drug in that class usually can be used.)

Common Gram-Positive Organism	# Isolates Tested (not all tested for each drug)	Penicillins and Cephalosporins					Macrolides		Fluoroquinolones			Amino-glycosides		Others (in alphabetical order)								
		Penicillin	Ampicillin	Amoxicillin / Clavulanate	Oxacillin	Ceftriaxone	Azithromycin	Erythromycin	Ciprofloxacin	Levofloxacin	Moxifloxacin	Gentamicin (do not use alone)	Gentamicin Synergy	Clindamycin	Daptomycin	Linezolid	Nitrofurantoin (for urine infections)	Quinupristin/ Dalfopristin	Rifampin (do not use alone)	Tetracycline	Trimethoprim / Sulfamethoxazole	Vancomycin
Inpatient																						
S. aureus (total)	604			66	66	66		49	68	71	83	98		71	99	100	100*	100	98	93	98	100
S. aureus (MRSA only)	203			0	0	0		16	29	31	55	97		58	98	99	*	100	98	90	95	100
S. aureus (MSSA only)	401			100	100	100		66	87	91	96	99		77	100	100	*	100	98	95	100	100

Staph coag. neg.	218			47	47		46		40	67	67	77	82		64	100	99	*	99	98	83	69	100
Strep pneumoniae	28*	50**		100*			96**	57*	57*	100*					89*						93*	82*	100*
Viridans strep group	47	94	94				94	47	53	98					91						69		100
Enterococcus faecalis	207	100	100							76	82		76			100	99	100			24		98
Enterococcus faecium	74	14	16							5	7		99			82	95	48*			30		36

Table 13.3

Common Organisms in Hospitals and Associated Antibiotic Coverage

Organism	Common coverage

Gram positive
– Cocci
  • In clusters – Staph
  • In chains – Strep
	– Penicillin
	– Cephalosporins (1st and 2nd generation)
	– Macrolides
	– Quinolones
	– Vancomycin (MRSA)
	– Bactrim
	– Clindamycin
	– Tetracyclines (Doxycycline)
	– Linezolid (MRSA, VRE)

Gram negative
– Cocci
  • Neisseria
– Coccobacillary
  • H. influenza
  • Moraxella
  • Acinetobacter
– Rods/bacilli
  • E. coli
  • Klebsiella sp.
  • Serratia marcescens
  • Proteus
	– Penicillin-beta lactams
	  (piperacillin-tazobactam)
	– Cephalosporins (3rd, 4th,5th generations)
	– Macrolides (Azithromycin)
	– Quinolones
	– Monobactams (Aztreonam)
	– Bactrim
	– Carbapenems
	– Aminoglycosides

– Anaerobic coverage (aspiration pneumonia, upper GI perforation)	– Metronidazole – Clindamycin – Broad-spectrum penicillin (such as Zosyn) – Fluoroquinolones – Carbapenems
– Atypical community-acquired pneumonia coverage	– Macrolides (legionella, mycoplasma, chlamydia) – Tetracyclines (rickettsia, chlamydia) – Quinolones (legionella, mycoplasma, chlamydia) – Ampicillin (listeria)
– Pseudomonas coverage (HAP, COPD, cystic fibrosis)	– Cephalosporins (some 3rd, 4th, 5th generation) (e.g., ceftazidime) – Carbapenems (e.g., meropenem) – Fluoroquinolones (Cipro, Levaquin) – Aminoglycosides

COPD, chronic obstructive pulmonary disease; HAP, hospital-acquired pneumonia; MRSA, methicillin-resistant *Staphylococcus aureus*; VRE, vancomycin-resistant enterococcus.

Table 13.4

Antibiotic Coverage by Organism

Gram-positive cocci				Gram-negative bacilli			Gram-negative cocci		Anaerobes	Atypicals
MRSA	MSSA	Streptococci	Enterococci	EKP*	Pseudomonas	ESC**	N. gonorrhea	N. meningitis		
		Penicillin								
	Oxacillin									
			Ampicillin IV/Amoxicillin PO					Amp/Amox		
	Cefazolin/cephalexin			Cefaz/cephalex						
	Cefoxitin			Cefoxitin					Cefoxitin	
	Ceftriaxone			Ceftriaxone						
	Cefepime					Cefepime				
	Unasyn IV/Augmentin PO			Piperacillin/tazobactam					Unasyn/AU:	
	Meropenem					Meropenem		AU		
						Ciprofloxacin				

(continued)

Table 13.4

Antibiotic Coverage by Organism (continued)

Gram-positive cocci			Enterococci	Gram-negative bacilli			Gram-negative cocci		Anaerobes	Atypicals
MRSA	MSSA	Streptococci		EKP*	Pseudomonas	ESC**	N. gonorrhea	N. meningitis		
		Levofloxacin				Levofloxacin				Levofloxacin
	Clindamycin				Centamycin/tobramycin				Above the diaphragm	
		Azithromycin								Azithromycin
		Vancomycin								
Doxycycline								Doxycycline		Doxycycline
TMP/SMZ (Bactrim)				TMP/SMZ		TMP/SMZ		TMP/SMZ	GI tract metronidazole	

*EKP = E. coli, Klebsiella, Proteus.

**ESC = Enterobacter, Serratia, Citrobacter.

MRSA, methicillin-resistant *Staphylococcus aureus*; MSSA, methicillin-sensitive *Staphylococcus aureus*; SMZ, sulfamethoxazole; TMP, trimethoprim.

to treating suspected or diagnosed CDI is to stop any antibiotics, if at all possible, and start empiric antibiotics.

1. Initial CDI: Oral vancomycin or fidaxomicin is recommended over metronidazole.
   a. Vancomycin 125 mg PO 4 ×/day × 10 days *OR*
   b. Fidaxomicin 200 mg PO BID × 10 days
   c. If vancomycin or fidaxomicin is not available, then use metronidazole 500 mg PO three times per day for 10 days.
2. Fulminant CDI, previously referred to as severe, complicated CDI, is characterized by shock, hypotension, ileus, or megacolon. Oral or rectal vancomycin and IV metronidazole are recommended.
   a. Vancomycin 500 mg PO Q 6 hours; if ileus is present, give vancomycin per rectum (PR) 500 mg in 100 mL normal saline Q 6 hours.
   b. Metronidazole 500 mg IV Q 8 hours.
   c. Consult surgical team for possible surgical management.
3. First recurrence:
   a. If metronidazole was first line of therapy, then use oral vancomycin × 10D.
   b. If oral vancomycin was first line of therapy, then use oral vancomycin as a tapered and pulsed regimen. Tapered and pulsed dosing example: After the initial dosage of 125 mg 4 times per day for 10 to 14 days, vancomycin dose remains the same and the frequency is reduced to 2 times per day for a week, then once per day for a week, and then once every 2 or 3 days for 2 to 8 weeks *OR*
   c. Treat with fidaxomicin 10-day course.
4. Greater than one recurrence: Use oral vancomycin as a tapered and pulsed regimen as described in 3b.
5. Fecal microbiota transplant should be considered for patients with multiple recurrences of CDI who have failed multiple courses of antibiotics.

Endocarditis

Endocarditis treatment depends on the type of valve, native versus prosthetic valve, and the type of organism and their resistance patterns. Following are the most common organisms and respective treatment options per IDSA guidelines. Please read the header carefully. Consult infectious disease team while the patient is admitted, as these patients will need outpatient follow-up. For patients who are hemodynamically unstable due to valvular dysfunction, consult the cardiac surgery team.

Infective endocarditis (IE) of native valve in penicillin-susceptible *Streptococcus viridans*:

- Penicillin G sodium 12 to 18 million units per 24 hours IV continuous infusion or divided doses Q 4 or 6 hours for 4 weeks *OR* Ampicillin 2 gm IV Q 4 hours if penicillin shortage exists *OR*
- Ceftriaxone 2 gm IV Q 24 hours for 4 weeks *OR*
- Penicillin G sodium 12 to 18 million units per 24 hours IV continuous infusion or divided doses Q 6 hours for 2 weeks *OR*
- Ceftriaxone 2 gm IV every 24 hours for 2 weeks *PLUS*
- Gentamicin sulfate 3 mg/kg IV or IM Q 24 hours for 2 weeks (C or 8th cranial nerve function). Peak goals 3 to 4 mcg/mL and trough goal <1 mcg/mL *OR*
- For patients unable to tolerate penicillin or ceftriaxone: vancomycin 30 mg/kg Q 24 hours in 2 equally divided doses for 4 to 6 weeks. Trough goal is 10 to 15 mcg/mL.

IE of native valve for relatively penicillin-resistant *Streptococcus viridans*:

- Penicillin G sodium 24 million units per 24 hours IV continuous infusion or divided doses Q 4 or 6 hours for 2 weeks *OR* ampicillin 2 gm IV Q 4 hours if penicillin shortage exists *OR* ceftriaxone 2 gm IV every 24 hours for 4 weeks if susceptible *PLUS*
- Gentamicin sulfate 3 mg/kg IV or IM Q 24 hours for 2 weeks.
  - **Note:** Gentamicin should not be used with patients with creatinine clearance <20 mL/min or 8th cranial nerve function.) Peak goals 3 to 4 mcg/mL and trough goal <1 mcg/mL.
- For patients unable to tolerate penicillin or ceftriaxone: vancomycin 30 mg/kg Q 24 hours in 2 equally divided doses for 4 weeks. Trough goal is 10 to 15 mcg/mL.

IE of a prosthetic valve due to penicillin-susceptible strain (<0.12 mcg/mL): *Streptococcus viridans*:

- Penicillin G sodium 24 million units Q 24 hours continuous infusion or in divided doses Q 4 to 6 hours for 6 weeks *OR* ceftriaxone 2 gm IV Q 24 hours IV or IM for 6 weeks.
- With or without gentamicin 3 mg /kg Q 24 hours IV or IM for 2 weeks.
- For patients unable to tolerate penicillin or ceftriaxone: vancomycin 30 mg/kg Q 24 hours in 2 equally divided doses for 6 weeks. Trough goal is 10 to 15 mcg/mL.

IE of a prosthetic valve due to relatively or fully penicillin-resistant strain (>0.12 mcg/mL): *Streptococcus viridans*:

- Penicillin G sodium 24 million units Q 24 hours continuous infusion or in divided doses Q 4 to 6 hours for 6 weeks *OR* ceftriaxone 2 gm IV Q 24 hours IV or IM for 6 weeks *PLUS*
- With or without gentamicin 3 mg/kg Q 24 hours IV or IM for 6 weeks (**Note:** Gentamicin should not be used with patients with creatinine clearance <20 mL/min.)

- For patients unable to tolerate penicillin or ceftriaxone: vancomycin 30 mg/kg Q 24 hours in 2 equally divided doses for 6 weeks. Trough goal is 10 to 15 mcg/mL.

For IE of native valve due to oxacillin-susceptible strains of staphylococci:

- Nafcillin or oxacillin 12 gm per 24 hours in 4 to 6 divided doses for 6 weeks *OR*
- Penicillin-allergic patients (nonanaphylaxis reactions): cefazolin 2 gm IV Q 8 hours for 6 weeks.

For IE of native valve due to oxacillin-resistant strains of staphylococci

- Vancomycin 30 mg/kg Q 24 hours in 2 equally divided doses for 6 weeks. Trough goal is 10 to 15 mcg/mL *OR*
- Daptomycin ≥8 mg/kg/dose for 6 weeks.

IE of a prosthetic valve due to oxacillin-susceptible strains of staphylococci:

- Nafcillin or oxacillin 12 gm per 24 hours in 4 to 6 divided doses for ≥6 weeks *PLUS*
- Rifampin 300 mg IV or PO Q 8 hours for 6 weeks *PLUS*
- Gentamicin 3 mg/kg Q 24 hours IV or IM in 2 or 3 divided doses for 2 weeks.

IE of a prosthetic valve due to oxacillin-resistant strains of staphylococci:

- Vancomycin 30 mg/kg Q 24 hours in 2 equally divided doses for ≥6 weeks. Trough goal is 10 to 15 mcg/mL.
- Rifampin 300 mg IV or PO Q 8 hours for ≥6 weeks *PLUS*
- Gentamicin 3 mg/kg Q 24 hours IV or IM in 2 or 3 divided doses for 2 weeks.
- **Note:** Do not use rifampin as a single agent; must use only in combination with another antibiotic, as rifampin is additive staph coverage. If used alone, patient will develop resistance.

IE of native or prosthetic valve due to penicillin and gentamicin-susceptible enterococcus:

- Ampicillin 2 gm IV Q 4 hours for 4 to 6 weeks *OR*
- Penicillin G sodium 18 to 30 million units Q 24 hours either continuously or in 6 equally divided doses for 4 to 6 weeks *PLUS*
- Gentamicin 3 mg/kg ideal body weight Q 24 hours IV or IM in 2 or 3 divided doses for 4 to 6 weeks *OR* for patients with creatinine clearance <50 mL/min:
- Ampicillin 2 gm every 4 hours for 6 weeks *PLUS*
- Ceftriaxone 2 gm IV every 12 hours for 6 weeks.
- For organisms resistant to penicillin, aminoglycosides, or vancomycin, consult infectious disease team.

IE of native or prosthetic valve due to HACEK organisms (Haemophilus spp., Aggregatibacter spp., *Cardiobacterium hominis, Eikenella corrodens,* and *Kingella* spp.):

- Ceftriaxone 2 gm IV or IM daily for 4 weeks for native valves and 6 weeks for prosthetic valves *OR*
- Ampicillin sodium 2 gm IV Q 4 hours for 4 weeks for native valves and 6 weeks for prosthetic valves *OR*
- Ciprofloxacin 500 mg Q 12 hours orally or 400 mg IV Q 12 hours for 4 weeks for native valves and 6 weeks for prosthetic valves.

Intraabdominal infections—watch for new guidelines emerging from IDSA.

- Obtain source control (drainage or surgical intervention) in addition to prescribing antimicrobials.
- Common first line:
  - Ceftriaxone (Rocephin) *OR* cefuroxime *OR* cefotaxime *PLUS* metronidazole (Flagyl) *OR*
  - Piperacillin/tazobactam (Zosyn) *OR*
- Second line:
  - Piperacillin/tazobactam (Zosyn) *OR*
  - Ceftazidime *OR* cefepime *PLUS* metronidazole (Flagyl)
  - Carbapenems (ertapenem, meropenem, imipenem/cilastatin)
- Third line (for hospital-acquired infections or when resistance occurs):
  - Consider ID consultation *PLUS*
  - Meropenem *OR* imipenem/cilastatin *OR*
  - Tigacycline *OR*
  - Ceftazidime/avibactam (Avycaz) *AND* metronidazole (Flagyl) *OR*
  - Gentamicin *OR* tobramycin or amikacin *AND* metronidazole (Flagyl) (Obtain ID consultation for aminoglycosides.)

Meningitis

When meningitis is suspected, immediate lumbar puncture should be completed along with blood cultures. The lumbar puncture should help determine whether the symptoms are bacterial or viral in nature, but will take time to get results, or the results may be inconclusive. Meningitis can be community acquired or healthcare acquired.

- For all patients with suspected bacterial meningitis, dexamethasone 10 mg IV Q 6 hours should be started either immediately before or concurrently with antibiotics.

Initial first line empiric treatment of community-acquired meningitis in an immunocompetent patient includes:

- Ceftriaxone 2 mg IV Q 12 hours *OR*
- Cefotaxime 2 gm IV Q 4 to 6 hours *PLUS*

- Vancomycin 15 to 20 mg/kg IV Q 8 to 12 hours (maximum 2 gm per dose or total daily dose of 60 mg/kg). Trough goal is 15 to 20 mg/L *PLUS*
- Ampicillin 2 gm IV Q 4 hours for patients over age 50 *PLUS*
- Acyclovir 10 mg/kg IV Q 8 hours for empiric viral encephalitis coverage (herpes simplex virus).

Initial empiric treatment of community acquired meningitis in an immunocompromised patient, initial empiric treatment includes:

- Vancomycin 15 to 20 mg/kg IV Q 8 to 12 hours (maximum 2 gm per dose or total daily dose of 60 mg/kg). Trough goal is 15 to 20 mg/L *PLUS*
- Ampicillin 2 gm IV Q 4 hours for patients over age 50 *PLUS*
- Cefepime 2 gm IV Q 8 hours *OR*
- Meropenem 2 gm IV Q 8 hours. If meropenem is used, then ampicillin is not needed, as it also covers listeria.
- Acyclovir 10 mg/kg IV Q 8 hours for empiric viral encephalitis coverage (herpes simplex virus).

Healthcare-associated meningitis and ventriculitis, empiric antibiotics should include:

- Vancomycin 15 to 20 mg/kg IV Q 8 to 12 hours (maximum 2 gm per dose or total daily dose of 60 mg/kg). Trough goal is 15 to 20 mg/L *PLUS*
- An antipseudomonal beta-lactam, such as cefepime, ceftazidime, or meropenem:
  - Cefepime 2 gm IV Q 8 hours *OR*
  - Ceftazidime 2 gm IV Q 8 hours *OR*
  - Meropenem 2 gm IV Q 8 hours.
- For patients with anaphylaxis to beta-lactam antimicrobial or if meropenem is contraindicated, aztreonam or ciprofloxacin is recommended for gram-negative coverage.
- For patients who are colonized or infected elsewhere with an antimicrobial-resistant organism, adjust the empiric regimen to cover these pathogens.
- Consider intraventricular antibiotics in patients who respond poorly to systemic antibiotics.
- Duration of treatment is 10 to 14 days, although some experts recommend gram-negative be treated up to 21 days.

Uncomplicated cystitis, pyelonephritis UTI, and catheter-associated UTI—watch for new guidelines emerging from IDSA.

Skin and Soft-Tissue Infections (SSTI)

For purulent furuncle, carbuncle, or abscess:

- Mild—Incision and drainage (I&D)

- Moderate: I&D, culture and sensitivities *PLUS* empiric treatment with Bactrim or doxycycline
- Culture and sensitivity results:
  - MRSA: sulfamethoxazole/trimethoprim (Bactrim)
    - Assess for allergy or sensitivity to sulfa with Bactrim
    - Monitor kidney function.
  - MSSA: dicloxacillin or cephalexin
- Severe: I&D, culture and sensitivities, *PLUS* empiric treatment with vancomycin *OR* daptomycin *OR* linezolid *OR* telavancin *OR* ceftaroline.
  - For daptomycin: Obtain CPK levels and monitor, as CPKs can increase with use.
  - Culture and sensitivity results:
    - MSSA: nafcillin *OR* cefazolin *OR* clindamycin
    - MRSA: vancomycin,dDoxycycline, Bactrim

For nonpurulent cellulitis and necrotizing infections:

- Mild: oral penicillin VK *OR* cephalosporin *OR* dicloxacillin *OR* clindamycin
- Moderate: IV penicillin *OR* ceftriaxone *OR* cefazolin *OR* clindamycin *PLUS* consider adding vancomycin for empiric MRSA coverage
- Severe:
  - Rule out necrotizing process with CT scan and emergent surgical inspection/debridement.
  - Empiric treatment: vancomycin*PLUS*S piperacillin-tazobactam
  - Culture and sensitivity results:
    - *Streptococcus pyogenes*: penicillin *PLUS* clindamycin
    - Clostridial spp.: penicillin *PLUS* clindamycin
    - Vibrio vulnificus: doxycycline *PLUS* ceftazidime
    - *Aeromonas hydrophila*: doxycycline *PLUS* ciprofloxacin
    - Polymicrobial: vancomycin *PLUS* piperacillin-tazobactam

Pneumonia

Classic signs of pneumonia include: fever, chills, cough, sputum production, hypoxia and/or increased oxygen requirements. Community acquired pneumonia (CAP) can be diagnosed within 48 hours of admission to the hospital, whereas hospital acquired pneumonia (HAP) is diagnosed after 48 hours of hospitalization or within 48 hours after discharge from a hospital stay of two days or more. Ventilator associated pneumonia (VAP) is diagnosed after 48 hours after intubation or within 48 hours after extubation when the patient was ventilated for 48 hours or more. Treatments for CAP, HAP and VAP are reviewed in Exhibit 13.2.

Exhibit 13.2

185

Treatment of Pneumonia

CAP

Outpatient treatment of CAP

No comorbidities or risk factors for MRSA or pseudomonas

– Amoxicillin or

– Doxycycline or

– Macrolide (if local pneumococcal resistance is <25%)

– Note: Amoxicillin and doxycycline do not cover pseudomonas.

With comorbidities (chronic heart, lung, liver, or renal disease; diabetes mellitus; alcoholism; malignancy; or asplenia) or risk factors for MRSA or pseudomonas.

– Combination therapy with amoxicillin/clavulanate or cephalosporin AND a macrolide or doxycycline

OR

– Monotherapy with respiratory fluoroquinolone

Inpatient Treatment of CAP

Nonsevere Inpatient CAP

– Standard therapy = Beta-lactam PLUS macrolide or respiratory fluoroquinolone.

– Prior MRSA = Standard therapy PLUS MRSA coverage AND obtain MRSA nasal swab, de-escalate if negative.

– Prior *Pseudomonas aeruginosa* = Standard therapy PLUS add coverage for *P. aeruginosa*, obtain respiratory cultures and de-escalate as able.

Severe Inpatient CAP

– Standard therapy = Beta-lactam PLUS macrolide OR beta-lactam PLUS respiratory fluoroquinolone.

– Prior MRSA = Standard therapy PLUS MRSA coverage and obtain MRSA nasal swab, and de-escalate if negative.

– Prior *Pseudomonas aeruginosa* = Standard therapy PLUS add coverage for *P. aeruginosa*, obtain respiratory cultures, and de-escalate as able.

KEY:

Beta-lactam:	• Ampicillin + sulbactam 1.5–3 g every 6 hours *OR* • Cefotaxime 1–2 g every 8 hours *OR* • Ceftriaxone 1–2 g daily *OR* • Ceftaroline 600 mg every 12 hours.
Macrolide:	• Azithromycin 500 mg daily *OR* • Clarithromycin 500 mg twice daily.
Respiratory Fluoroquinolone	• Levofloxacin 750 mg daily *OR* • Moxifloxacin 400 mg daily.
MRSA coverage:	• Vancomycin (15 mg/kg every 12 hours, adjust based on trough goal 15–20) *OR* • Linezolid (600 mg every 12 hours).
Pseudomonas coverage:	• Piperacillin-tazobactam (4.5 g every 6 hours) *OR* • Cefepime (2 g every 8 hours) *OR* • Ceftazidime (2 g every 8 hours) *OR* • Imipenem (500 mg every 6 hours) *OR* • Meropenem (1 g every 8 hours) *OR* • Aztreonam (2 g every 8 hours).

(continued)

Exhibit 13.2

Treatment of Pneumonia (*continued*)

HAP

Empiric antibiotic therapy for hospital-acquired pneumonia

Not at high risk of mortality and no factors increasing the likelihood of MRSA.
One of the following:
– Piperacillin-tazobactam 4.5 g IV q6h
OR
– Cefepime 2 g IV q8h
– Levofloxacin 750 mg IV daily

OR
– Imipenem 500 mg IV q6h
– Meropenem 1 g IV q8h

Not at high risk of mortality but with factors increasing the likelihood of MRSA.
One of the following:
– Piperacillin-tazobactam 4.5 g IV q6h
– Cefepime or ceftazidime 2 g IV q8h
OR
– Levofloxacin 750 mg IV daily
– Ciprofloxacin 400 mg IV q8h
OR
– Imipenem 500 mg IV q6h
– Meropenem 1 g IV q8h
OR
– Aztreonam 2 g IV q8h
PLUS
– Vancomycin 15 mg/kg IV q8–12h with goal to target 15–20 mg/mL trough level
  (consider a loading dose of 25–30 mg/kg × one for severe illness)
OR
– Linezolid 600 mg IV q12h

High risk of mortality or intravenous antibiotics within 90 days, prescribe two of the following, and while avoiding double beta-lactam coverage.
– Piperacillin-tazobactam 4.5 g IV q6h
OR
– Cefepime or ceftazidime 2 g IV q8h
OR
– Levofloxacin 750 mg IV daily
– Ciprofloxacin 400 mg IV q8h
OR
– Imipenem 500 mg IV q6h
– Meropenem 1 g IV q8h
OR
– Amikacin 15–20 mg/kg IV daily
– Gentamicin 5–7 mg/kg IV daily
– Tobramycin 5–7 mg/kg IV daily
OR
– Aztreonam 2 g IV q8h

(continued)

Exhibit 13.2

Treatment of Pneumonia (*continued*)

PLUS

– Vancomycin load with 25 mg/kg IV × 1 then 15 mg/kg IV q8–12h with target trough of 15–20 mg/mL

OR

– Linezolid 600 mg IV q12h

If MRSA coverage is not needed, be sure to include coverage for MSSA, including piperacillin-tazobactam, cefepime, levofloxacin, imipenem, meropenem.

VAP

Empiric treatment options for suspected HAP/VAP when MRSA and double antipseudomonal/gram-negative coverage are needed.

Choose one from A, B, and C:

A. (Gram + coverage with MRSA coverage):

– Vancomycin load 25 mg/kg IV × 1, then 15–20 mg/kg Q 8–12h, trough goal 15–20.

OR

– Linezolid 600 mg IV or PO Q 12h

AND

B. (Gram – coverage with antipseudomonal coverage with beta-lactam based agents)

– Piperacillin-tazobactam 4.5 gm IV Q 6h or via extended infusions over 4 hours Q 8h

OR

– Cefepime 2 g IV q8h

– Ceftazidime 2 g IV q8h

OR

– Imipenem 500 mg IV q6h

– Meropenem 1 g IV q8h

OR

– Aztreonam 2 g IV q8h

AND:

C. (Gram – coverage with antipseudomonal coverage with non-beta-lactam based agents)

– Ciprofloxacin 400 mg IV q8h

– Levofloxacin 750 mg IV q24h

OR

– Amikacin 15–20 mg/kg IV q24h

– Gentamicin 5–7 mg/kg IV q24h

– Tobramycin 5–7 mg/kg IV q24h

Note: Be sure to renal dose based on patient's creatinine clearance. If in doubt, consult a pharmacist.

ANTIBIOTIC STEWARDSHIP

Antibiotic stewardship is every prescriber's responsibility to minimize antibiotic resistances. Hospitals are required to have a dedicated antibiotic stewardship program, including physicians, other prescribers, pharmacists, and patients on the team. The core components of hospital antibiotic stewardship programs include:

Table 13.4

Comparison of risk factors for *Pseudomonas aeruginosa* infection vs. MDRO *Pseudomonas aeruginosa* infection:	
Risk factors for *Pseudomonas aeruginosa* infection	**Risk factors for multidrug-resistant *Pseudomonas aeruginosa* infections:**
– Known pseudomonas colonization – IV antibiotics within 90 days – Frequent chronic obstructive pulmonary disease exacerbations requiring glucocorticoid and/or antibiotic use – Other structural lung disease (e.g., bronchiectasis or cystic fibrosis) – Immunosuppression	– Previous hospital or ICU admission within the last year – Prior penicillin, cephalosporins, carbapenem, or fluoroquinolone use – Higher illness severity scores

- Hospital leadership commitment, including human, financial, and information technology support.
- Accountability by appointing a designated leader responsible for the management of the program and outcomes.
- Pharmacy expertise with the appointment of a pharmacist as a coleader of the program to aid in implementation efforts and antibiotic use.
- Action by using audit and feedback tools or requiring preauthorization to improve antibiotic use.
- Tracking or monitoring of antibiotic prescribing, the impact of interventions, and organism resistance patterns or *C. diff* infection rates.
- Reporting antibiotic use and resistance to prescribers, pharmacists, nursing, and leadership teams.
- Education of prescribers, pharmacists, nurses, and patients about adverse outcomes of antibiotics and optimal prescribing.

MULTIDRUG-RESISTANT ORGANISMS

Multidrug-resistant organisms (MDROs) continue to rise, causing nearly 3 million antibiotic-resistant infections in the United States each year, resulting in 35,000 deaths. Previous exposure to IV antibiotics is the primary factor giving rise to MDROs, especially with VAP. The number-one risk factor for MDR HAP, MDR MRSA HAP/VAP, and MDR pseudomonas HAP/VAP is prior IV antibiotic use within 90 days. Risk factors for MDROs associated with VAP include:

- use of intravenous antibiotics in the past 90 days
- ≥5 days of hospitalization prior to the occurrence of VAP

Table 13.5

Classifications of Resistance		
MDR	**XDR**	**PDR**
Isolate is not susceptible to at least 1 agent in ≥3 antimicrobial categories	Isolate is not susceptible to at least 1 agent in all but 2 or fewer antimicrobial categories	Not susceptible to any agents in any antimicrobial categories

MDR, multidrug-resistant; PDR, pandrug-resistant; XDR, extensively drug-resistant.

- septic shock at the time of VAP
- acute respiratory distress syndrome before VAP
- acute renal replacement therapy prior to VAP

Fast Facts

IV antibiotics within 90 days is the number-one risk factor for MDR HAP and VAP!

Drug resistance can escalate over time with exposure to multiple antibiotics. The more antibiotics an organism is exposed to, the more drugs it can become resistant to. Three categories define the extent of an organism's resistance to antibiotics (see Table 13.5).

The Centers for Disease Control and Prevention (CDC) ranks the seriousness of drug resistances. Four categories of threats have been defined, and organisms have been categorized on this living list. AG-ACNPs need to recognize the threat these organisms pose to patients and adopt antibiotic stewardship practices to prevent these lethal infections. Consider an infectious diseases consultation when these or other multidrug-resistant organisms are identified in the hospitalized populations.

1. Urgent threats
   a. Carbapenem-resistant *Acinetobacter*
   b. *Candida auris*
   c. *Clostridioides difficile* (*C. diff*)
   d. Carbapenem-resistant *Enterobacterales*
   e. Drug-resistant *Neisseria gonorrhoeae*
2. Serious threats
   a. Drug-resistant *Campylobacter*
   b. Drug-resistant *Candida*
   c. ESBL-producing *Enterobacterales*

d. Vancomycin-resistant *Enterococcus* (VRE)
e. Multidrug-resistant *Pseudomonas aeruginosa*
f. Drug-resistant Nontyphoidal salmonella
g. Drug-resistant *Salmonella* serotype Typhi
h. Drug-resistant shigella
i. Methicillin-resistant *Staphylococcus aureus* (MRSA)
j. Drug-resistant *Streptococcus pneumoniae*
k. Drug-resistant tuberculosis

3. Concerning threats
a. Erythromycin-resistant group A streptococcus
b. Clindamycin-resistant group B streptococcus

4. Watch List
a. Azole-resistant *Aspergillus fumigatus*
b. Drug-resistant *Mycoplasma genitalium*
c. Drug-resistant *Bordetella pertussis*

Fast Facts

The AG-ACNP should consider an infectious diseases consultation when multidrug-resistant organisms are identified in a hospitalized patient.

FUNGAL INFECTIONS

Invasive fungal infections (IFI) are less common than bacterial or viral infections, but pose great risk of morbidity and mortality to acutely and critically ill hospitalized patients. Fungal organisms are the third most common organism observed in ICU patients and the fourth most commonly identified pathogen causing nosocomial bloodstream infections. Candida species are the most common, and invasive aspergillosis is the second most common IFI in immunocompromised patients in ICU. Risk factors for invasive fungal infections include:

- peripheral and central intravenous catheters
- bladder catheters
- mechanical ventilation >10 days
- lack of enteral nutrition
- use of parenteral nutrition
- hospital-acquired bacterial infection
- cardiopulmonary bypass duration greater than 120 min
- diabetes mellitus
- APACHE II score >16
- major surgery

- fungal colonization
- acute renal failure requiring hemodialysis
- severe sepsis
- use of broad-spectrum antibiotics
- red cell transfusion

Diagnostic Testing for Fungal Infections Includes:

- The Fungitell® assay specifically detects (1–3)-beta-d-glucan found in the fungal cell wall of *Candida* species, *Pneumocystis jirovecii*, as well as *Aspergillus*, *Fusarium*, and *Acremonium* species.
- Galactomannan is a polysaccharide antigen found in the cell wall of aspergillus species. This test is specific to diagnose invasive aspergillosis.

IMMUNOCOMPROMISED PATIENTS

In patients who are immunocompromised, diagnosing and managing infections is a challenge. After recognizing who is immunocompromised, the next step is to determine what factors put them at risk for common and opportunistic infections as well as antibiotic resistances. Immunocompromised patients include those who are or have

- taken chronic steroids (>6 months),
- a current cancer or are receiving chemotherapy or radiation therapy,
- receiving immune modulating therapies (such as monoclonal antibodies),
- a history of splenectomy,
- transplant recipients on antirejection medications such as cyclosporine, mycophenolate, tacrolimus, and so forth,
- hepatic failure, or
- HIV/AIDS.

Immunocompromised patients commonly do not have classic signs of infection. They may not become febrile, tachycardic, tachypneic, or develop leukocytosis. Rather, they report vague symptoms, commonly stating, "I just don't feel well" or "I feel run down." The AG-ACNP must always have a high index of suspicion for infection in immunocompromised patients. Additionally, immunocompromised patients can acquire common and uncommon pathogens as well as MDROs and opportunistic infections. Examples include:

Fungal infections

- *Candida* species
- coccidiomycosis
- cryptococcus

Bacterial infections

- pneumocystis jirovecii pneumonia (PJP)
- mycobacterium tuberculosis
- mycobacterium avium complex

Viral infections

- cytomegalovirus (CMV) (especially in transplant patients)
- herpes simplex virus (HSV)

Parasites

- cryptosporidiosis
- toxoplasmosis

Fast Facts

Immunocompromised patients may not have classic signs of infection. Maintain a high index of suspicion for infection in this population, and have a lower threshold to obtain cultures and start antibiotics when their fever is 38.0 °C or 100.4 °F.

This chapter summarizes common organisms and infections and their associated anti-infective agents. Managing infections and their associated anti-infective agents is challenging for all nurse practitioners. The key is to keep building on your knowledge base, adding new data in small bits and pieces. Don't try to memorize all the organisms and all the antibiotics; rather, learn the organisms and treatments by source of the infection, such as lungs, central nervous system, urinary tract, or bowel. And then break it down by specific organisms and their sensitivities. When in doubt, ask questions and refer to infectious disease specialists.

References

Baddour, L. M., Wilson, W. R., Bayer, A. S., Fowler, V. G., Tleyjeh, I. M., Rybak, M. J., Barsic, B., Lockhart, P. B., Gewitz, M. H., Levison, M. E., Bolger, A. F., Steckelberg, J. M., Baltimore, R. S., Fink, A. M., O'Gara, P., & Taubert, K. A. (2015). Infective endocarditis in adults: diagnosis, antimicrobial therapy, and management of complications. *Circulation*, *132*(15), 1435–1486. https://doi .org/10.1161/CIR.0000000000000296

CDC. *Core Elements of Hospital Antibiotic Stewardship Programs*. U.S. Department of Health and Human Services. www.cdc.gov/antibiotic-use /core-elements/hospital.html

CDC. (2021, 2 March 2021). *2019 AR Threats Report*. www.cdc.gov/drugresistance /biggest-threats.html?CDC_AA_refVal=https%3A%2F%2Fwww.cdc .gov%2Fdrugresistance%2Fbiggest_threats.html

De Vlieger, G., Lagrou, K., Maertens, J., Verbeken, E., Meersseman, W., & Van Wijngaerden, E. (2011). Beta-d-glucan detection as a diagnostic test for invasive Aspergillosis in immunocompromised critically ill patients with symptoms of respiratory infection: an autopsy-based study. *Journal of Clinical Microbiology, 49*(11), 3783–3787. https://doi.org/10.1128/jcm.00879-11

Garner, D. (2019). *Nuts and Bolts of Microbiology: Key Concepts of Microbiology and Infection* (3rd ed.). www.cdc.gov/antibiotic-use/healthcare/pdfs /hospital-core-elements-H.pdf

Griffiths, M. J., McGill, F., & Solomon, T. (2018). Management of acute meningitis. *Clinical Medicine, 18*(2), 164–169. https://doi.org/10.7861 /clinmedicine.18-2-164

Kalil, A. C., Metersky, M. L., Klompas, M., Muscedere, J., Sweeney, D. A., Palmer, L. B., Napolitano, L. M., O'Grady, N. P., Bartlett, J. G., Carratalà, J., El Solh, A. A., Ewig, S., Fey, P. D., File, T. M. Jr., Restrepo, M. I., Roberts, J. A., Waterer, G. W., Cruse, P., Knight, S. L., & Brozek, J. L. (2016). Management of adults with hospital-acquired and ventilator-associated pneumonia: 2016 Clinical practice guidelines by the Infectious Diseases Society of America and the American Thoracic Society. *Clinical Infectious Diseases, 63*(5), e61–e111. https://doi.org/10.1093/cid/ciw353

Khilnani, G. C., Zirpe, K., Hadda, V., Mehta, Y., Madan, K., Kulkarni, A., Mohan, A., Dixit, S., Guleria, R., & Bhattacharya, P. (2019). Guidelines for antibiotic prescription in intensive care unit. *Indian Journal of Critical Care Medicine: Peer-Reviewed, Official Publication of Indian Society of Critical Care Medicine, 23*(Suppl. 1), S1–S63. https://doi.org/10.5005 /jp-journals-10071-23101

Magiorakos, A. P., Srinivasan, A., Carey, R. B., Carmeli, Y., Falagas, M. E., Giske, C. G., Harbarth, S., Hindler, J. F., Kahlmeter, G., Olsson-Liljequist, B., Paterson, D. L., Rice, L. B., Stelling, J., Struelens, M. J., Vatopoulos, A., Weber, J. T., & Monnet, D. L. (2012, 1 March 2012). Multidrug-resistant, extensively drug-resistant and pandrug-resistant bacteria: An international expert proposal for interim standard definitions for acquired resistance. *Clinical Microbiology and Infection, 18*(3), 268–281. https://doi .org/10.1111/j.1469-0691.2011.03570.x

McDonald, L. C., Gerding, D. N., Johnson, S., Bakken, J. S., Carroll, K. C., Coffin, S. E., Dubberke, E. R., Garey, K. W., Gould, C. V., Kelly, C., Loo, V., Shaklee Sammons, J., Sandora, T. J., & Wilcox, M. H. (2018). Clinical Practice guidelines for clostridium difficile infection in adults and children: 2017 update by the Infectious Diseases Society of America (IDSA) and Society for Healthcare Epidemiology of America (SHEA). *Clinical Infectious Diseases, 66*(7), e1–e48. https://doi.org/10.1093/cid/cix1085

Metlay, J. P., Waterer, G. W., Long, A. C., Anzueto, A., Brozek, J., Crothers, K., Cooley, L. A., Dean, N. C., Fine, M. J., Flanders, S. A., Griffin, M. R., Metersky, M. L., Musher, D. M., Restrepo, M. I., & Whitney, C. G. (2019). Diagnosis and treatment of adults with community-acquired pneumonia: An official clinical practice guideline of the American Thoracic Society and Infectious Diseases Society of America. *American Journal of Respiratory and Critical Care Medicine, 200*(7), e45–e67. https://doi.org/10.1164/rccm.201908-1581ST

Raman, G., Avendano, E. E., Chan, J., Merchant, S., & Puzniak, L. (2018, 4 July 2018). Risk factors for hospitalized patients with resistant or multidrug-resistant

Pseudomonas aeruginosa infections: A systematic review and meta-analysis. *Antimicrobial Resistance & Infection Control*, 7(1), 79. https://doi.org/10.1186/s13756-018-0370-9

Stevens, D. L., Bisno, A. L., Chambers, H. F., Dellinger, E. P., Goldstein, E. J., Gorbach, S. L., Hirschmann, J. V., Kaplan, S. L., Montoya, J. G., & Wade, J. C. (2014). Practice guidelines for the diagnosis and management of skin and soft tissue infections: 2014 Update by the Infectious Diseases Society of America. *Clinical Infectious Diseases*, 59(2), e10–e52. https://doi.org/10.1093/cid/ciu444

Tunkel, A. R., Hasbun, R., Bhimraj, A., Byers, K., Kaplan, S. L., Scheld, W. M., van de Beek, D., Bleck, T. P., Garton, H. J. L., & Zunt, J. R. (2017). 2017 Infectious Diseases Society of America's clinical practice guidelines for healthcare-associated ventriculitis and meningitis. *Clinical Infectious Diseases*, 64(6), e34–e65. https://doi.org/10.1093/cid/ciw861

Wunderink, R. G., Srinivasan, A., Barie, P. S., Chastre, J., Cruz, C. S. D., Douglas, I. S., Ecklund, M., Evans, S. E., Evans, S. R., Gerlach, A. T., Hicks, L. A., Howell, M., Hutchinson, M. L., Hyzy, R. C., Kane-Gill, S. L., Lease, E. D., Metersky, M. L., Munro, N., Niederman, M. S., Restrepo, M. I., Sessler, C. N., Simpson, S. Q., Swoboda, S. M., Guillamet, C. V., Waterer, G. W., & Weiss, C. H. (2020). Antibiotic stewardship in the intensive care unit: An Official American Thoracic Society Workshop Report in Collaboration with the AACN, CHEST, CDC, and SCCM. *Annals of the American Thoracic Society*, 17(5), 531–540. https://doi.org/10.1513/AnnalsATS.202003-188ST

Zhou, W., Li, H., Zhang, Y., Huang, M., He, Q., Li, P., Zhang, F., Shi, Y., & Su, X. (2017). Diagnostic value of galactomannan antigen test in serum and bronchoalveolar lavage fluid samples from patients with nonneutropenic invasive pulmonary Aspergillosis. *Journal of Clinical Microbiology*, 55(7), 2153–2161. https://doi.org/10.1128/JCM.00345-17

14

Endocrine Acute Care

The endocrine system can be confusing for many nurse practitioners. The pathophysiology and diagnostic interpretations can be challenging to commit to memory and are difficult to recall when needed in clinical situations. Many students memorize this information to successfully pass their academic exam and then rememorize for the national certification exam, only to realize that once in a great while the information is truly needed to care for a patient.

In this chapter, the reader will learn

- to differentiate between diabetic ketoacidosis and hyperglycemic hyperosmolar syndrome;
- to manage diabetic ketoacidosis and hyperglycemic hyperosmolar syndrome;
- to interpret thyroid testing;
- the signs, symptoms, and treatment of thyroid storm and myxedema coma; and
- how to interpret a cosyntropin stimulation test.

DIABETES MELLITUS

The most common endocrine disorder among acutely and critically ill patients, hyperglycemia is most commonly caused by physiological stress of acute or critical illness. In other words, the flight-or-fight response has been activated. Alternatively, the patient may have underlying uncontrolled or undiagnosed diabetes, has been noncompliant with medical management, or cannot afford prescribed medications. The severity of hyperglycemia is directly proportional to the severity of illness.

Criteria for Diagnosis of Diabetes Mellitus:

- Symptoms of DM plus random blood glucose ≥200 mg/dL
- Fasting plasma glucose ≥126 mg/dL
- Hemoglobin A1c ≥6.5%
- 2-hour glucose 200 mg/dL during an oral glucose tolerance test

Treatment Goals:

- HbA1c <7.0
- Preprandial capillary plasma glucose 80 to 130 mg/dL
- Postprandial capillary plasma glucose <180 mg/dL
- Blood pressure <140/90
- LDL <100

GLYCEMIC CONTROL

Glycemic control is considered a best practice for hospitalized patients. Leukocytes do not work as well in a hyperglycemic state. All hospitalized patients are at risk for infection, thus poor performance of leukocytes predisposes patients to worse outcomes.

Blood glucose goals for hospitalized patients can be conservative or liberal. Commonly hospitalized patient goals are <180 mg/dL. Populations that require special attention include:

- Hospitalized patients <180 mg/dL.
- Cardiothoracic surgery patients <120 mg/dL.
- For acutely neurologically impaired patients (traumatic brain, new stroke), keep blood glucose >100 mg/dL; avoid hypoglycemia to prevent secondary injury.

AG-ACNPs need to understand properties of the variety of insulin preparations, including onset and duration (see Tables 14.1 and 14.2). Additionally, AG-ACNPs commonly need to transition from insulin infusions to long acting insulin and sliding scales (see Table 14.3).

Fast Facts

Metformin is typically avoided in the inpatient setting, as it can cause high lactic acidosis in the setting of IV contrast. Hospitalized patients who decompensate may require CAT scans with contrast to diagnose or treat their conditions, thus it is best to avoid this agent in the inpatient setting.

DIABETIC CRISES

Two types of diabetic crises exist: diabetic ketoacidosis (DKA) and hypergylcemic hyperosmolar syndrome (HHS) (see Tables 14.4 and 14.5).

Table 14.1

Properties of Insulin Preparations

Preparation	Onset (hours)	Peak (hours)	Effective duration (hours)
Fast-acting			
Aspart	<.25	.5–1.5	2–4
Glulisine	<.25	.5–1.5	2–4
Lispro	<.25	.5–1.5	2–4
Short-acting			
Regular	<.5–1.0	2–3	3–6
Long-acting			
Degludec	1–9	–	42
Detemir	1–4	–	12–24
Glargine	2–4	–	20–24
NPH	2–4	4–10	10–16

NPH, ormal pressure hydrocephalus.

Table 14.2

Common Sliding Scale Insulin Regimens

	Low	Medium	High
<120	0 units	0 units	0 units
120–150	1 unit	2 units	3 units
151–200	2 units	4 units	6 units
201–250	3 units	6 units	9 units*
251–300	4 units	8 units*	12 units*
301–350	5 units	10 units*	15 units*
351–400	6 units	12 units*	*
>400 call NP**	**	**	**

*Consider adding or increasing long-acting insulin, initiate an insulin infusion, or add an oral agent if taking PO.
**Watch for DKA or HHS.
DKA, diabetic ketoacidosis; HHS, hyperglycemic hyperosmolar syndrome.

These crises can be accompanied by other types of acidosis that can confuse the picture. Starvation ketosis, alcoholic ketoacidosis and high anion gap acidosis can also be seen concomitantly, making the picture more difficult to differentiate from each other.

Table 14.3

	Transition from Insulin Infusions to Long-Acting Insulin	
	Patients who are eating meals	Patients who are on continuous tube feedings or stable parenteral nutrition
Step 1:	Calculate total dosage in 24 hours.	Calculate total dosage in 24 hours.
Step 2:	Provide 50% of total dose in long-acting formulation (if giving NPH insulin, divide this dose in half for a.m. and p.m. dosing).	Provide 75% of total dose in long acting formulation (if giving NPH insulin, divide this dose in half for a.m. and p.m. dosing).
Step 3:	Provide 25% of total dose in short-acting formulation scheduled with meals.	Provide insulin sliding scale Q6 hours.
Step 4:	Provide insulin sliding scale ac/hs or dose by carbohydrate intake.	Stop insulin drip 2 hours after long-acting dose given.
Step 5:	Stop insulin drip 1–4 hours after long-acting dose given (dose depends on type of long acting insulin given—see Table 14.1 for onset timing).	NOTE: If giving long-acting insulin and tube feeding will be off for >2 hours, be sure to hold the long-acting insulin or start a glucose-containing IV fluid to prevent hypoglycemia.

NPH, Normal pressure hydrocephalus.

Table 14.4

	Typical Presentation of Diabetic Crises	
	Diabetic Ketoacidosis (DKA)	Hyperglycemic Hyperosmolar Syndrome (HHS)
Typically affects:	DM Type I	Diabetes Type II
Onset	Hours	Days
Causes/ precipitating event	Insufficient insulin administration* Infection (pneumonia, UTI, cellulitis) Infarction (STEMI, CVA, Mesentery) Drugs (cocaine) Pregnancy	Concurrent with other illness Myocardial or cerebral ischemia Pancreatitis Corticosteroid use Diuretics
Symptoms	Nausea/vomiting Thirst/polydipsia Polyuria Abdominal pain	Polyuria Decreased PO intake Weight loss

(continued)

Table 14.4

Typical Presentation of Diabetic Crises (*continued*)

	Diabetic Ketoacidosis (DKA)	Hyperglycemic Hyperosmolar Syndrome (HHS)
Signs	Tachycardia	Profound dehydration
	Tachypnea/Kussmaul respirations	Confusion
	Ketosis (fruity breath)	Lethargy
	Abdominal pain (epigastric)	Coma
	Lethargy, obtundation	

*Can be iatrogenic in hospitalized patients if insulin is withheld in setting of being NPO for a procedure.

CVA, cerebrovascular accident; DKA, diabetic ketoacidosis; HHS, hyperglycemic hyperosmolar syndrome; NPO, nonprofit organization; STEMI, ST-elevation myocardial infarction; UTI, urinary tract infection.

Table 14.5

Laboratory Values at Presentation of Diabetic Crisis

	DKA	HHS
Glucose mg/dL	250–600	600–1,200
Sodium, meq/L	125–135	135–145
Potassium	Normal to increased	Normal
Creatinine	Slightly increased	Moderately increased
Osmolality mOsm/mL	300–320	330–380
Plasma ketones	++++	+/–*
Serum bicarbonate meq/L	<15	Normal to slightly decreased
Arterial pH	6.8–7.3	>7.3
Arterial PaCO2 mmHg	20–30	35–45
Anion Gap	increased	Normal to slightly increased

*May have ketonuria secondary to starvation.

DKA, diabetic ketoacidosis; HHS, hyperglycemic hyperosmolar syndrome.

Management of Diabetic Ketoacidosis

Step 1: Replace fluids:

2 to 3 L of .9% normal saline (NS) over first 1 to 3 hours

- 10 to 20 mL/kg per hour,
- then .45% NS at 250 to 500 mL/hr,
- change to D5%1/2NS solution when glucose <250 mg/dL at 150 to 250 mL/hr.

Step 2: Assess and treat potassium level:

> If potassium is <3.3 mmol/L, begin potassium repletion. Do not administer insulin until potassium is corrected.

Step 3: Administer short-acting insulin:

> Bolus .1 units/kg IV × 1, then start insulin infusion at .1 units /kg; increase two- to three-fold if no response by 2 to 4 hours.

Fast Facts

Bicarbonate is not recommended for management of acidosis in DKA as long as the pH is >7.0.

Step 4: Identify precipitating event:

> Initiate workup to identify precipitating event (e.g., EKG/troponin, infection workup, blood cultures, urinalysis, chest x-ray, pregnancy test, assess for trauma and noncompliance).

Step 5: Reassess:

> Check glucose every 1 hour.
> Check basic metabolic profile, including anion gap every 4 hours for first 24 hours.
> Monitor urine output.

Step 6: Ongoing electrolyte repletion and wean insulin drip as glucose comes down.

Step 7: End points of resuscitation:

> Continue above until glucose is 150 to 200 mg/dL and acidosis has resolved/anion gap is closed. Patient will begin to feel better and become hungry. Once they are eating, administer long-acting insulin and allow drip to overlap 2 to 4 hours.

Step 8: Obtain endocrine consult for comanagement and/or outpatient follow-up of diabetic crisis.

Fast Facts

HHS management is similar, except much larger volumes of fluids are required, as patients are more severely dehydrated and require less insulin.

Corrected Serum Sodium Calculations

Sodium level is frequently falsely low in the setting of severe hyperglycemia, thus calculating a corrected serum sodium level is useful to manage fluids in DKA and HHS. The formula to calculate CNa is:

- Na in mEq/L + .016(glucose in mg/dL − 100)
- In an example of a patient with a Na level of 140 and glucose of 600, the calculations would look like this:

- Na of 140 + .016(glucose of 600 − 100) = CNa
- 140 + .016(500) = CNa
- 140 + 8 = CNa 148

Estimating Free Water Deficit

To obtain accurate free water deficit, first calculate the corrected serum sodium level. The formula to calculate the free water deficit is:

- .6(weight in kg) ([CNa − 140]/140)
- Example: For a 100 kg person with a CNa level of 148, the calculations would look like this:
  - .6(100) ([148 − 140]/140) = Free water deficit in liters
  - 60(8/140) = 3.43 L of free water deficit.

Fast Facts

Identifying the causative factor of DKA ensures timely and proper treatment of the often-serious underlying reason and prevention of recurrence and readmission. Infection is the number-one trigger of DKA.

HYPOGLYCEMIA

Severe hypoglycemia can be neurologically devastating to acutely and critically ill patients (see Table 14.6).

Table 14.6

Common Causes of Hypoglycemia	
Insulin mediated	**Noninsulin mediated**

• Oral diabetic secretagogue medications
    ◦ Glyburide
    ◦ Glipizide
    ◦ Glimepiride
    ◦ Gliclazide
    ◦ Repaglinide
 • Exogenous insulin—iatrogenic
 • Postgastric bypass hypoglycemia
 • Insulinoma
 • Antibody-mediated
 • Noninsulinoma pancreatogenous hypoglycemia
 • Genetic mutations
	• Critical illness
	    ◦ End-stage hepatic or renal failure
	    ◦ Late stages of sepsis
	    ◦ Severe malnutrition
	 • Adrenal insufficiency
	 • Non-islet cell tumor
	 • Toxins
	    ◦ Alcohol
	    ◦ Salicylate
	 • Medications
	    ◦ Fluoroquinolones
	    ◦ Lithium
	    ◦ Indomethacin
	    ◦ Quinine
	    ◦ Pentamidine
	    ◦ Propoxyphene

Preventable Iatrogenic Causes of Hypoglycemia

The primary cause of iatrogenic hypoglycemia is associated with use of insulin drips and/or concurrent cessation of a source of glucose administration. Three specific examples of iatrogenic hypoglycemia to avoid:

- A patient receives their home dose of long- and short-acting insulin and then is made NPO for a procedure.
- A patient is receiving multiple infusions of sedatives, analgesics, and insulin. The patient requires a bolus of analgesics and the insulin infusion is erroneously bolused rather than the analgesic agent.
- A patient is receiving long-acting insulin and continuous tube feedings. The tube feeding is stopped at the time of discharge to a skilled nursing facility or rehabilitation. Upon arrival at the institution, there is often a lag time until the tube feeding is restarted. This has been known to cause severe and catastrophic results. To avoid, transport patient on a dextrose infusion and continue until tube feeding is started.

THYROID DISORDERS

Thyroid stimulating hormone (TSH) is commonly abnormal in acute and critical illness states (sick euthyroid syndrome). Administration of thyroid hormone in the setting of sick euthyroid syndrome during acute and critical illnesses does not improve patient outcomes. Review outpatient records for results within the last 3 months, unless you believe the thyroid disease is the primary problem. Interpretation of TSH is inversely proportional; in other words, a high TSH means the thyroid is not producing hormones normally (see Figure 14.1).

Thyroid Storm

Thyroid storm is the most severe form of hyperthyroidism and can present with a variety of signs and symptoms, including hyperpyrexia, diaphoresis, thyroid nodule or enlargement, ophthalmopathy, tachycardia, atrial fibrillation or other tachyarrhythmias, congestive heart failure, nausea, vomiting diarrhea, severe abdominal pain, jaundice, hepatosplenomegaly/vascular congestion, pretibial edema, anxiety, psychosis, seizure, and hyperreflexia.

Management always includes an endocrinology consult. Other treatment options include inhibiting synthesis of T_3 and T_4 with methimazole 20 to 30 mg Q6 hours or propylthiouracil (PTU) 200 to 400 mg PO Q4 to Q6 hours, which has more side effects. Blockade of T_3 and T_4 release with saturated solution of iodine (SSKI) up to 5 drops Q8 hours after antithyroid medication started. Blockade peripheral conversion of T_4 to T_3 with hydrocortisone 100 mg Q8 hours or dexamethasone 4 mg Q12

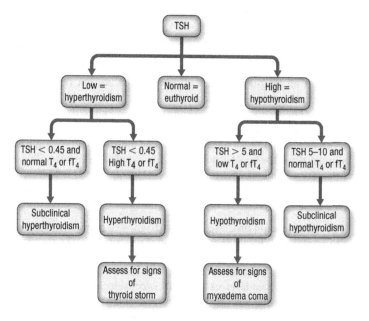

Figure 14.1 Interpretation of TSH in absence of acute or critical illness.

Key: fT_4 = Free T_4

hours. Block hormone action on target organs with propanolol 1 mg IV loading dose, then 60 to 80 mg PO Q4 to Q6 hours. Alternatively, an esmolol infusion can be used for it's ease of titration.

Myxedema Coma

Myxedema coma is the most severe form of hypothyroidism. Classic signs and symptoms include hypothermia, goiter, periorbital edema, goiter, edema of tongue and pharynx, hypoventilation and hypoxemia, diaphragmatic weakness, aspiration events, pleural effusions, bradycardia, dilated cardiomyopathy, prolonged QT, pericardial effusion, ileus, megacolon, ascites, somnolence, lethargy, depression, coma, seizures, and dry, coarse skin/hair.

Management always includes endocrinology consultation and administration of levothyroxine (T_4). Start with a loading dose of 200 to 250 mcg IV. Follow with a weight-based daily dose starting 24 hours later. For older adults or those with cardiovascular disease, forgo the loading dose to prevent complications. Improvement is typically seen in 1 to 3 days. If hypothermic, use passive rewarming rather than active rewarming. Treat with corticosteroids until adrenal insufficiency is ruled out.

ADRENAL INSUFFICIENCY

Two common situations in which adrenal insufficiency occurs in hospitalized patients are when

1. a patient on long-term glucocorticoid therapy has not received this intervention while hospitalized;
2. a patient has been acutely or critically ill for a prolonged period of time and has adrenal dysfunction from ischemia, injury, hemorrhage, or other sequela of critical illness. This can be more difficult to diagnose, as many times the hypotension can be attributed to the primary illness. Consider adrenal insufficiency if vasopressor support is not weaning off 2 to 3 days after initiation of treatment for the underlying condition (see Table 14.7).

Two main thought processes exist to diagnose adrenal insufficiency due to acute and critical illness in hospitalized patients. The first is to perform a random cortisol test and treat based on these results, and the other practice is to perform a cosyntropin stimulation test.

A random cortisol level <23.4 µg/dL is considered adrenally insufficient; if >23.4 µg/dL, it is considered normal. Some providers round up to 25 or down to 20 or even 18 to determine whether to treat or not. If the result falls within the 25 to 18 range, a cosyntropin stimulation test can be performed to further aid in the diagnosis.

Cosyntropin Stimulation Test:

1. Draw random or baseline cortisol level.
2. Administer 1 mcg (low dose) or 250 mcg (high dose) of cosyntropin (ACTH).
3. Draw cortisol level 30 minutes after cosyntropin administered.
4. Draw cortisol level 60 minutes after cosyntropin administered.

Table 14.7

Signs and Symptoms of Adrenal Insufficiency	
Glucocorticoid Deficiency	**Mineralocorticoid**
• Fatigue	• Dizziness
• Anorexia	• Hypotension/orthostatic hypotension
• Abdominal pain	• Hyponatremia
• Nausea/vomiting	• Hyperkalemia
• Myalgia	
• Hypotension	
• Anemia	
• Hypercalcemia	
• Hypoglycemia	

Interpretation: An increase of 9 points from baseline is positive for the patient to respond. A patient with a response <9 is considered a nonresponder who requires treatment with either hydrocortisone 50 mg IV Q6 hours or 100 mg IV Q8 hours. Providers will typically see vasopressor requirements decreasing after the second dose.

References

Annane, D., Pastores, S. M., Rochwerg, B., Arlt, W., Balk, R. A., Beishuizen, A., Briegel, J., Carcillo, J., Christ-Crain, M., Cooper, M. S., Marik, P. E., Umberto Meduri, G., Olsen, K. M., Rodgers, S., Russell, J. A., & Van den Berghe, G. (2017, 1 December 2017). Guidelines for the diagnosis and management of critical illness–related corticosteroid insufficiency (CIRCI) in critically ill patients (Part I): Society of Critical Care Medicine (SCCM) and European Society of Intensive Care Medicine (ESICM) 2017. *Intensive Care Medicine*, *43*(12), 1751–1763. https://doi.org/10.1007/s00134-017-4919-5

Gosmanov, A. R., Gosmanova, E. O., & Kitabchi, A. E. (2018). Hyperglycemic crises: Diabetic ketoacidosis (DKA), and hyperglycemic hyperosmolar state (HHS). In K. R. Feingold, B. Anawalt, A. Boyce et al. (Eds.), Endotext [Internet]. MDText.com, Inc. www.ncbi.nlm.nih.gov/sites/books/NBK279052

Hudson, M. S., McMahon, G. T. (2017). Glycemic emergencies. In S. J. McKean, J. J. Ross, D. D. Dressler, & D. B. Scheurer (Eds.), *Principles and Practice of Hospital Medicine* (2nd ed., pp. 1171–1177). McGraw Hill Education.

Mooradian, A. D. (2018). Evidence-based management of diabetes in older adults. *Drugs & Aging, 35*(12), 1065–1078.

15

Musculoskeletal and Integumentary Acute Care

AG-ACNPs will encounter patients with life-threatening illness or injury related to the musculoskeletal or integumentary systems. Rapid identification and management are essential to preserving limb and life. Being able to communicate findings to the consulting teams by using accurate terminology and descriptions is critical. This chapter reviews dermatology terminology and associated life-threatening skin disorders that AG-ACNPs may encounter.

In this chapter, you will learn

- to accurately assess muscle strength,
- diagnose and treat compartment syndrome,
- dermatology terminology,
- to differentiate between cellulitis and necrotizing fasciitis,
- common drugs that cause Stevens–Johnson syndrome (SJS) and toxic epidermal necrolysis (TEN),
- types of burns and fluid resuscitation, and
- airway management of thermal burns.

STRENGTH

Older hospitalized patients can lose an average of 5% of muscle mass daily. Refer to Table 15.1 for strength grading. Early mobilization maintains prehospital mobility, flexibility, and functional capacity. Additionally, early mobilization promotes independence, increases

Table 15.1

Muscle Strength Grading Scale	
0	No muscle movement
1	Palpable or visible muscle contraction only
2	Active movement with gravity eliminated
3	Active movement against gravity
4	Active movement against gravity and provides some resistance
5	Active movement against gravity with normal resistance
NT	Unable to exert effort or muscle unavailable due to immobilization, pain, or contractures, and so forth

NT, not tested.

appetite and mood, reduces atelectasis, decreases the incidence of delirium, and reduces ventilator days and hospital length of stay. Thus, it's critical, especially for older patients, to minimize bed rest and mobilize the patient as soon as possible to promote an optimal outcome.

COMPARTMENT SYNDROME

Compartment syndrome (CS) of the extremity commonly occurs in patients with traumatic extremity injuries or burns. CS is a surgical emergency requiring rapid diagnosis and intervention to salvage the limb. Patients at risk for compartment syndrome include those with

- tibial fractures,
- open fractures of long bones,
- traumatic vascular injuries, and
- those who are found down after prolonged downtime and have had an extremity compressed, causing ischemia.

CS occurs due to lack of blood flow to the affected extremity. The lack of blood flow causes ischemia, which leads to edema, which leads to further ischemia and further edema, which leads to a vicious cycle of perpetual ischemia threatening the viability of the extremity. AG-ACNPs must maintain a high index of suspicion for CS in patients with these injuries.

In early stages, patients may complain of paresthesia or weakness. Patients commonly develop exquisite and increasing pain that is refractory to analgesics. Severe pain, disproportionate with exam, is the hallmark sign of CS. Additionally, passive stretching of the extremity will significantly increase pain. A physical exam may reveal full, tight compartments but is not consistent for all patients. Obtain compartment pressures to diagnose CS. Stat surgical consultation for fasciotomies is required to preserve the function and viability of the extremity. Necrotic tissue may require debridement. Anticipate that viable muscles will swell and may be managed with negative pressure wound therapy until either primary closure or skin grafting can be performed.

Fast Facts

Maintain a high index of suspicion for compartment syndrome in patients with tibial fractures, open fracture of long bones and vascular injuries to extremities. Observe for the six Ps of a threatened extremity: pain, pallor, paresthesia, paralysis, poikilothermia, and pulselessness. Pulselessness is a late finding!

DERMATOLOGY TERMINOLOGY

Use correct terminology to describe a rash or skin lesion to accurately and concisely communicate when consulting a dermatologist (see Table 15.2). Providing an accurate description, along with clinical

Table 15.2

Dermatology Terminology

Terms	
Macule	a flat spot <5 mm in diameter
Patch	a flat spot >5 mm in diameter
Plaque	a flat-topped raised lesion
Papule	a rounded raised lesion (a bump)
Nodule	raised lesion >.5 cm
Vesicle	a small blister
Bulla	a large blister
Erosion/ulcer	localized loss of epidermis/dermis
Descriptors	
Color	Color is critical to the description. Describe the color of the lesion or rash (e.g., erythematous, purpuric, violaceous, hyper-pigmented, hypopigmented, depigmented, black [necrotic])
Distributions	Does the lesion or rash form a pattern (e.g., localized, symmetric, acral, central, sun-protected, sun-exposed, and so forth)?
Configurations	Does the lesion or rash follow any configuration (e.g., linear, annular, dermatomal, serpiginous, grouped, isolated, scattered, targetoid, and so forth)?

status (e.g., fever, hypotension) aids them in determining the urgency of the consult and prioritizing their time should it be a dermatological emergency.

SKIN SOFT-TISSUE INFECTIONS

AG-ACNPs will frequently manage skin and soft-tissue infections (SSTIs). And occasionally AG-ACNPs will encounter dermatological emergencies, including necrotizing fasciitis, Stevens–Johnson syndrome (SJS), toxic epidermal necrolysis (TEN), or vascular diseases. Differentiating between these can be challenging. The difference between cellulitis and a dermatologic emergency is the presence of fever and rash, blistering or skin sloughing, widespread skin involvement, and involvement of mucous membranes. Definitive diagnosis and management should include consultation with both the dermatology team and either the burn team or plastics and reconstructive surgery team.

Cellulitis

Cellulitis is defined as infection and inflammation involving the dermis and subcutaneous tissues. *Staphylococcus aureus* is responsible for most cases of cellulitis. Signs include erythema, edema, induration, warmth to touch, pain at site, and may or may not include purulent drainage or fever. Abscesses or furuncles may form with pain and tenderness as the primary findings, and palpation may reveal fluctuance. Abscesses require incision and drainage. All skin and soft-tissue infections require systemic antibiotics. Hospitalization should be considered in patients who present with fever, pain, rapidly advancing erythema; patients who failed oral therapy, have significant comorbid conditions such as peripheral vascular disease, diabetes, immunocompromised states; and patients who exhibit signs of septic shock such as tachycardia, tachypnea, hemodynamic instability or elevated lactic acid level.

Necrotizing Fasciitis

Necrotizing fasciitis (NF) is a rapidly progressive infection involving the subcutaneous structures and fascia. Fournier gangrene is a form of NF affecting the genitals and perineum. NF commonly occurs in diabetics; older patients; patients with cardiovascular diseases, including peripheral vascular disease; and individuals who abuse alcohol. NF can develop from infected hair follicles, after surgical intervention, or after traumatic injuries and commonly affects the abdominal wall and extremities. Infectious etiology includes group A streptococcus (most common), *Staphylococcus aureus*, *Enterococci*, *E. coli*, *Pseudomonas*, *Bacteroides*, and *Clostridium* species. Early skin changes are similar to cellulitis, including erythema, edema, and tenderness. Within 24 to 36 hours, color can change to dusky gray-blue and bullae can form. Patients may also develop crepitus from gas gangrene in the affected tissues. Patients then develop symptoms of sepsis and can progress rapidly into septic shock. X-rays or CT scans should be done to assess for gas tracking along the fascia. Treatment is immediate surgical consultation with emergent surgical debridement in an operating room. Antibiotic therapy should include

- one agent to inhibit protein synthesis and toxin production; clindamycin is commonly used. Linezolid or aminoglycosides can also be effective;
- one agent with activity against MRSA, such as vancomycin, daptomycin, ceftaroline, or linezolid;
- one agent active against gram-negative rods and anaerobes, such as a fourth-generation cephalosporin, piperacillin-tazobactam, or a carbapenem.

Anticipate admission to ICU for septic shock, and follow the sepsis management algorithm. Serial debridement is typically required. Intravenous immune globulin (IVIG) can be used to neutralize streptococcal toxins and thus may improve mortality in patients with streptococcal infections. Morbidity is common, including loss of extremity function and disfiguration, depending on the extent of the tissue requiring debridement. Mortality is 20% to 40%.

OTHER DERMATOLOGICAL EMERGENCIES

Stevens–Johnson Syndrome, Toxic Epidermal Necrolysis

STS and TEN are caused by a hypersensitivity reaction to a medication or infection that leads to apoptosis of keratinocytes. These syndromes cause full-thickness necrosis of skin and mucosal surfaces. TEN is about 95% medication related, including antibiotics, anticonvulsants, allopurinol, and NSAIDs. SJS is about 50% medication related or infection related. Onset of SJS and TEN is typically within 1 to 3 weeks of medication initiation and may have flu-like prodrome before the skin is affected. Mucosal changes occur in nearly 90% of cases and begin with pharyngitis, cheilitis, and conjunctivitis and may progress to blisters and sloughing. Treatment includes stopping the causative agent or treating the precipitating infection (see Table 15.3). Optimal management should occur in a burn unit, where ideal fluid management can occur and ophthalmology consultation can be obtained. Complications include sepsis, AKI, pneumonia, pneumonitis, acute respiratory distress syndrome (ARDS), and GI bleeding. Mortality is 5% to 30%. Patients may be left with permanent pigmentary changes, hair loss, and nail damage.

Table 15.3

Drugs Associated with SJS and TENS

Strongly associated	Associated	Suspected
• Allopurinol	• Diclofenac	• Pantoprazole
• Lamotrigine	• Doxycycline	• Glucocorticoids
• Sulfamethoxazole	• Amoxicillin/ampicillin	• Omeprazole
• Carbamazepine	• Ciprofloxacin	• Tetrazepam
• Phenytoin	• Levofloxacin	• Dipyrone (metamizole)
• Nevirapine	• Amifostine	• Terbinafine
• Sulfasalazine	• Oxcarbazepine	• Levetiracetam
• Sulfonamide	• Rifampin	
• Oxicam NSAIDs		
• Phenobarbital		

NSAIDs, nonsteroidal anti-inflammatory drugs; SJS, Stevens–Johnson syndrome; TENS, toxic epidermal necrolysis.

BURNS

Burn patients have unique needs requiring multidisciplinary care to achieve positive outcomes. A tertiary care healthcare system is well positioned to coordinate the enormous resources, including acute, chronic, and rehabilitative care. Refer patients to a higher level of care for burns with partial thickness (second degree); burns greater than 10% of the total body surface area (TBSA); burns of the face, hands, feet, genitals, perineum, or across major joints; and burns with full thickness (third degree) of any size.

Types of burns AG-ACNPs may encounter include thermal burns and electrical burns. Additionally, burn patients may have other concomitant injuries, depending on the mechanism of the burn (e.g., motor vehicle crash). A systematic assessment and evaluation of a patient with thermal burns starts with the primary survey.

Primary Survey

1. Airway management
   a. Assess for supraglottic injury (edema) from thermal injury; singed facial hair, carbonaceous sputum, soot in/near the mouth, hoarseness, stridor, increased work of breathing, inability to manage secretions.
   b. Manage with early intubation or tracheostomy.
2. Breathing and ventilation
   a. assess ability to oxygenate and ventilate; circumferential burns of the neck and chest require bedside escharotomy.

3. Circulation and cardiac status
   a. Tachycardia 100 to 120 is common with catecholamine release. Fluid management should be based on weight and burn size. Evaluate the perfusion on all extremities, especially those with circumferential burns. Loss of pulses is a late finding. An escharotomy is indicated for impaired perfusion in a circumferentially burned extremity.
4. Disability, neurologic deficit, and gross deformity
   a. Change in mental status can be due to other injuries, hypoxia, hypotension/shock, or preexisting condition.
5. Exposure
   a. Completely undress the patient and examine for injuries while maintaining a warm environment to prevent hypothermia.

Fast Facts

Patients with airway edema, singed facial hair, carbonaceous sputum, soot in the mouth and airways, hoarseness, stridor, increased work of breathing, or inability to manage secretions should be intubated immediately.

Secondary Survey

Upon completion of the primary survey, immediately perform the secondary survey to assess for other injuries. Secondary assessment includes assessment of extent of burns; laboratory values, including carboxyhemoglobin levels to assess for carbon monoxide; x-rays; CT scans; and so forth. Evaluation of TBSA burned is commonly calculated based on the rule of nines (see Figure 15.1 and Table 15.4).

Fluid Resuscitation

Fluid resuscitation should be initiated promptly and customized based on patient needs. Avoid over- or underresuscitation for good outcomes. Underresuscitation can lead to shock and organ failure, whereas overresuscitation can lead to compartment syndromes (both abdominal and extremity) and respiratory compromise, including ARDS. Parkland and modified Brooke formulas can be used to calculate fluid needs, which typically range from 2 to 4 mL/kg/% burn over 24 hours. Fluids should be lactated Ringer solution.

- Parkland formula: 4 mL/kg/% burn—half is given in first 8 hours, and half over the next 16 hours.
- Modified Parkland formula: 3 to 4 mL/kg/% burn—half is given in first 8 hours, and half over the next 16 hours.
- Modified Brooke formula: 2 mL/kg/% burn—half is given in first 8 hours, and half over the next 16 hours.

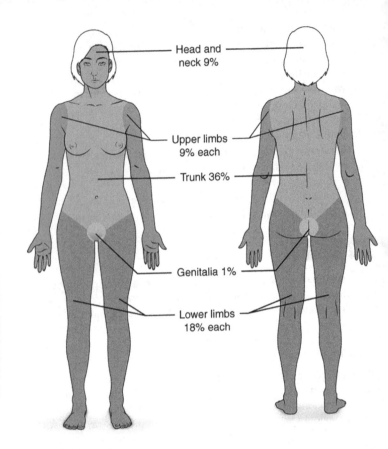

Figure 15.1 Rule of nines.

Resuscitation goal is to titrate fluids to obtain urine output (UOP) of .3 to .5 mL/kg/hr for adults. Patients with inhalation injuries, electrical burns, and delayed resuscitation commonly have increased fluid needs, in which case the AG-ACNP should monitor for increased intraabdominal hypertension and abdominal compartment syndrome. Management after the first 24 hours and beyond commonly includes albumin in the ongoing resuscitation.

Fast Facts

Optimal fluid resuscitation of burn patients is essential to avoid deleterious effects. Resuscitation goal is to titrate fluids to maintain UOP .3 to .5 mL/kg/hr. Overresuscitation can lead to compartment syndrome and ARDS. Underresuscitation can lead to shock and organ failure.

Table 15.4

Burn Classification

Depth	Level of injury	Clinical features	Treatment/Outcome
Superficial (1st degree)—not included when calculating burn size	Epidermis	Erythema (dry, pink to red, sunburn-like), mild edema, no blisters, blanches, painful	Healing in 3–6 days, no scarring
Superficial partial thickness (2nd degree)	Papillary dermis	Blisters, moist, weeping, pink to red underlying tissue; mild to moderate edema; blanches; severe pain	Healing in 7–21 days; hypertrophic scar rare; return to full function
Deep partial thickness (deep 2nd degree)	Reticular dermis	Red to white; moderate edema; blisters rare, wet or waxy, dry; decreased pain sensation; pain present to deep pressure	Healing in 2–6 weeks; possible surgical excision and grafting; scars common if not grafted; earlier return to function with surgery
Full thickness (3rd degree)	Hypodermis	Waxy white to leathery dry and inelastic; no blanching; severe edema; no blisters; absent pain sensation; pain present in surrounding areas of second-degree burn	Weeks to months to heal; requires surgical excision and grafting; scarring; functional limitation more common if not grafted
Deep full thickness (4th degree)	Involves fascia and muscle and/or bone	Insensate, black eschar formation, no edema or blisters, no pain	Healing time is weeks to months; grafts required

Airway Management

Elevated carboxyhemoglobin levels should be managed with supplemental FiO_2. Upper-airway burns should keep the head of bed (HOB) greater than 30 degrees to prevent further airway edema. Ongoing assessment of hoarseness, shortness of breath, increased work of breathing, use of accessory muscles, and hypoxia are signs of respiratory failure. Patients who require intubation are at risk for developing ARDS. As such, they should be managed with protective lung strategies, including low tidal volumes and close monitoring of plateau pressures.

Wound Care

Partial-thickness burns and skin graft donor sites benefit from occlusive dressings for longer periods (minimally one week). Heat-preserving dressings are recommended to prevent contamination, dryness, and evaporation from the wound. If these are not available, then use moist dressings. Leaving the dressing on for as long as possible provides the best chance for healing. An important factor in choosing a dressing is the amount of exudate from the wound. Ongoing consultation with the burn team and/or plastic and reconstructive surgery teams for initial and ongoing debridement as well as wound-care treatments is essential.

Nutrition

Nutrition is a critical element for burn patients who have higher-than-normal caloric requirements and are at high risk for malnutrition. Burn patients have a metabolic response to the burn, which includes hypermetabolism, increased protein catabolism, and weight loss. The extent of this hypercatabolism is nearly proportional to the percent of the burn. Malnutrition can impair wound healing, maintenance of muscle strength, and the immune system. Adults with >20% TBSA need a high-protein diet of 1.5 to 2 g protein/kg/d. Early nutrition should be started as soon as possible. Conventional oral nutrition is preferred, with enteral tube feedings preferred over parenteral nutrition. Many patients are not able to sufficiently supplement their diet to meet the caloric needs, thus supplemental tube feedings may be essential to meet the nutritional needs of the patient.

Rehabilitation

Burn patients commonly need rehabilitation, especially to treat the contractile forces of scarring. Treatment is especially necessary for burns across joints, including the neck, shoulders, elbows, wrist and hand, hip, knee, and foot/ankle. Early consultation of physical therapy (PT) and occupational therapy (OT) is essential to secure splints to preserve function and range of motion.

Electrical Injuries

Electrical injuries are rare but life-threatening. There are two categories of electrical injuries: low-voltage injuries (LVI) are those with <1,000 volts, and high-voltage injuries (HVI) with >1,000 volts. LVI can also cause severe damage depending on the electrical field, amperage, and duration of contact with the source. HVI typically causes high temperatures in tissues, which leads to more extensive tissue injury and causes microvascular coagulation. LVI causes less tissue damage but more commonly produces cardiac arrhythmias, including sinus tachycardia, premature ventricular contractions, ventricular tachycardia, and ventricular fibrillation. The burns are typically the most severe at the entry point and exit point. Both cause muscular necrosis, causing rhabdomyolysis, which if not treated promptly may lead to acute kidney injury requiring dialysis; compartment syndrome requiring fasciotomies; and if severe enough, amputation.

The history of present illness should include the voltage, type of current (AC or DC), amperage, and duration of contact. Workup of electrical injuries includes complete blood count (CBC), electrolytes, creatinine levels, urinalysis, serum myoglobin, arterial blood gas if patient is in rhabdomyolysis, creatinine kinase-MB (CK-MB), and troponin. ECGs are warranted if any chest pain or arrhythmia is noted. Additional x-rays or CT scans are ordered depending on how the electrical current traveled through the body.

Management, as with thermal burns, requires assessment of airway, breathing, circulation, deformity, and exposure. Electrical injuries should be on telemetry for the first 24 to 48 hours. Those with significant burns should receive IV fluid resuscitation to maintain UOP .5 to 1 mL/kg/hr. Alkalization of the urine with sodium bicarbonate infusion can be helpful, as can diuresis to maintain UOP. Consult nephrology for potential for hemodialysis (HD) or continuous renal replacement therapy (CRRT) if the patient becomes oliguric.

Long-term sequelae of electrical injury include neurological symptoms and deficits such as headaches, weakness, neuropathy, paresthesia, loss of balance, ataxia, seizures, and syncope. Physical sequelae include pain and fatigue. Musculoskeletal sequelae include weakness, contractures, muscle spasms, decreased range of motion, and limited mobility. Amputations may be required for high-voltage injuries. Psychological symptoms include memory or attention deficits, irritability, depression and/or posttraumatic stress disorder.

Fast Facts

All burn patients should receive an updated tetanus vaccination.

In summary, the musculoskeletal and integumentary systems can present emergent conditions the AG-ACNP must be able to diagnose and intervene upon. Patients can either present with or develop compartment syndrome and skin and soft-tissue infections while hospitalized. Burn patients present a complex problem requiring specialized care; however, they can present at any facility, requiring the AG-ACNP to stabilize and transfer to a burn center, or the AG-ACNP may work in a tertiary care trauma and burn center. Regardless, the AG-ACNP must be familiar with the diagnosis and treatment of burn victims.

References

Ahuja, R. B., Gibran, N., Greenhalgh, D., Jeng, J., Mackie, D., Moghazy, A., Moiemen, N., Palmieri, T., Peck, M., & Serghiou, M. (2016). ISBI practice guidelines for burn care. *Burns*, *42*(5), 953–1021.

Ashbaugh, C. (2017). Skin and soft-tissue infections. In S. J. McKean, J. J. Ross, D. D. Dressler, & D. B. Scheurer (Eds.), *Principles and Practice of Hospital Medicine* (pp. 1582–1588). McGraw Hill Education.

Drew, J. M., Demos, H. A., & Pellegrini, V. D. (2017). Management of common perioperative complications in orthopedic surgery. In S. J. McKean, J. J. Ross, D. D. Dressler, & D. B. Scheurer (Eds.), *Principles and Practice of Hospital Medicine* (2nd ed., pp. 437–446). McGraw Hill Education.

Zemaitis, M. R., Foris, L. A., Lopez, R. A., & Huecker, M. R. (2020). Electrical injuries. In *StatPearls [Internet]*. StatPearls Publishing. www.ncbi.nlm.nih .gov/books/NBK448087

III

Special Populations

16

Patients With Substance-Use Disorders and Toxicological Issues

AG-ACNPs regularly encounter patients with substance-use disorders, toxic ingestions, and overdoses, including both intentional and unintentional overdoses. Additionally, alcohol-use disorder and its associated withdrawal symptoms and delirium tremens complicate and prolong hospital courses. Additionally, many hospitalized patients undergo conscious sedation and may become overmedicated. The AG-ACNP must be able to promptly recognize oversedation and rescue the patient with the proper antidote.

In this chapter, you will learn

- terminology associated with opioid use,
- the components of SBIRT,
- to compare and contrast toxidromes,
- antidotes and adult dosing for a variety of toxins, and
- signs of serotonin syndrome and common causative agents.

OPIOID-USE DISORDERS

The response to the opioid epidemic has heightened awareness and broadened insights into acute and chronic pain management and the consequences of opioid misuse. AG-ACNPs should use contemporary terminology to accurately diagnose, treat, and document a patient's pain conditions and conditions associated with opioid use.

- **Acute pain**—Abrupt onset of pain with a known cause, such as an injury or surgery. Typically improves as the body heals and has a duration of <3 months.
- **Chronic pain**—Pain that lasts >3 months; can be caused by a disease, inflammation, injury, or medical treatment.
- **Acute on chronic pain**—A new acute pain that occurs simultaneously with a chronic pain. Requires supplemental/additive interventions to address both the acute and chronic pain.
- **"Opiates" versus "opioids":** Although these terms are often used interchangeably, they are different:
  - **piates:** refer to natural opioids such as heroin, morphine, and codeine.
  - **pioids:** refer to all natural, semisynthetic, and synthetic opioids.
- **Tolerance:** Repeated use of a drug reduces response to the drug.
- **Physical dependence:** Adaptation to a drug which, when stopped, produces symptoms of withdrawal.
- **Opioid-use disorder:** A problematic pattern of opioid use that causes significant impairment or distress. Diagnosis is based on specific criteria including, but not limited to, inability to cut down or control use, and use that results in social problems and/or failure to satisfy work, school, or home obligations. The term *opioid-use disorder* is preferred over other similar terms, including *opioid abuse, opioid dependence,* or *opioid addiction.*
- **Drug misuse:** The use of illegal drugs and/or the use of prescription drugs in a manner other than as directed by a doctor, such as use in greater amounts, more often, taking a drug longer than directed, or using someone else's prescription.

Screening, Brief Intervention, and Referral to Treatment

Use of the Screening, Brief Intervention, and Referral to Treatment (SBIRT) approach is essential to quality care. This tool is designed to evaluate both alcohol and drug use. The components of SBIRT, as the name indicates, are screening, brief intervention, and referral to treatment. These three steps are outlined as follows.

Screening

All patients should be screened to identify unhealthy use of alcohol and drugs. Seventy-five percent to 85% of individuals will screen negative. Perform the AUDIT-C tool to assess alcohol use (see Tables 16.1 and 16.2) and the single-item drug screen to assess drug use (see Tables 16.3 and 16.4). Patients who screen positive are at high risk for acute consequences such as trauma and/or illness. Risky drinking is considered:

a. For healthy men up to age 65: >4 drinks/day AND >14 drinks/week.
b. For all healthy women and men over 65: >3 drinks/day AND 7 drinks/week.

Table 16.1

AUDIT-C Tool to Assess Alcohol Use						
	0	1	2	3	4	Score
How often do you have a drink containing alcohol?	Never	Monthly or less	2–4 ×/ month	2–3 ×/ week	≥4 ×/ week	
How many drinks containing alcohol do you have on a typical day when you are drinking?	1–2	3–4	5–6	7–9	≥10	
How often do you have five or more drinks on one occasion?	Never	<Monthly	Monthly	Weekly	Daily	

Scoring: Positive score = women ≥3; men ≥4. If positive, assess with full audit.
If negative, reinforce healthy decisions and continue with drug screening.
If AUDIT-C is positive, assess for alcohol-use severity with AUDIT tool in Table 16.3.

Table 16.2

AUDIT Tool for Alcohol Severity						
	0	1	2	3	4	Score
Carry AUDIT-C score over:						
How often during the last year have you found that you were not able to stop drinking once you had started?	Never	<Monthly	Monthly	Weekly	Daily, or near daily	
How often during the last year have you failed to do what was expected of you because of drinking?	Never	<Monthly	Monthly	Weekly	Daily, or near daily	
How often during the last year have you needed a drink first thing in the morning to get yourself going after a heavy drinking session?	Never	<Monthly	Monthly	Weekly	Daily, or near daily	

(continued)

Table 16.2

AUDIT Tool for Alcohol Severity (*continued*)

	0	1	2	3	4	Score
How often during the last year have you had a feeling of guilt or remorse after drinking?	Never	<Monthly	Monthly	Weekly	Daily, or near daily	
How often during the last year have you been unable to remember what happened the night before because of your drinking?	Never	<Monthly	Monthly	Weekly	Daily, or near daily	
Have you or someone else been injured because of your drinking?	No		Yes, not in the last year		Yes, within the last year	
Has a relative, friend, doctor, or other healthcare worker been concerned about your drinking or suggested you cut down?	No		Yes, not in the last year		Yes, within the last year	

Scoring: <13 Women or <15 men = risky use.
≥13 women or ≥15 men = need further diagnostic evaluation and referral.

Table 16.3

Single-Item Drug Screen

Question	How many times in the past year have you used an illegal drug or used a prescription medication for nonmedical purposes?
Scoring	>1 is positive for both men and women. If positive, perform DAST-10 in Table 16.4 to assess severity of drug use.

Fast Facts

All patients should be screened to identify unhealthy use of alcohol and drugs, regardless of age, race, gender, or socioeconomic status.

Table 16.4

DAST-10 for Drug-Use Severity

Have you used drugs other than those required for medical reasons? (Carry screening score over as *yes*.)	0	1
Do you use >1 drug at a time?	No	Yes
Are you always able to stop using drugs when you want to?	No	Yes
Have you ever had blackouts or flashbacks as a result of drug use?	No	Yes
Do you ever feel bad or guilty about your drug use?	No	Yes
Does your spouse (or parents) ever complain about your involvement with drugs?	No	Yes
Have you neglected your family because of your use of drugs?	No	Yes
Have you engaged in illegal activities in order to obtain drugs?	No	Yes
Have you ever experienced withdrawal symptoms when you stopped taking drugs?	No	Yes
Have you had medical problems as a result of your drug use?	No	Yes

Note: All patients receiving DAST-10 should receive a brief intervention.
Scoring: ≥3 women and men = further diagnostic evaluation and referral warranted.

Table 16.5

Brief Intervention Steps and Suggested Dialogue

Brief intervention steps	Suggested dialogue
Understand the patient's perspective of use	"I'd like to know more about your use of [X]." "Help me understand what you enjoy about using [X]?" "What do you regret about using [X]?"
Give information and feedback	"Is it OK if we review some of the health risk of using [X]?" If yes, "Which ones are you aware of?" If not, indicate problems and consequences.
Enhance motivation to change	"Are you ready to make a change in your use of [X]?" "On a scale of 0–10, how ready are you to change any aspect of your use of [X]?" (10 = fully ready; 0 = not at all ready)
Give advice and negotiate goal	"What can you do to stay healthy and safe?" "Where do you go from here?"

1. **Brief intervention:** For those with positive screens, a brief intervention (BI) is completed to provide feedback about the unhealthy substance use. It is designed to increase awareness of the risks associated with the behavior. This should be a collaborative conversation to enhance the patient's motivation to change their alcohol and/or other drug use to lower their risk for alcohol- and drug-related problems (see Table 16.5).

2. **Referral to treatment:** About 5% of people screened will need referral. The referral increases access to addiction assessment and treatment. For inpatients, consult social work and, if available, addiction medicine services. Discharge options include referral to acute treatment services if medical intervention is needed to manage withdrawal symptoms; clinical stabilization services for those who have already been detoxified or do not require medical supervision; or provide local outpatient contact numbers to Alcoholics Anonymous or Narcotics Anonymous for peer support and Al-Anon for family groups.

TOXIDROMES

A toxidrome is a cluster of signs and symptoms that are classically associated with exposure to a substance or category of substances (see Table 16.6).

Opioids and Sedatives

Hospitalized patients can develop over-sedation or overdose, as they are commonly prescribed narcotics, benzodiazepines, muscle relaxants, and other agents that can impair cognitive functions. Additionally, many patients receive conscious sedation or general anesthetics for invasive or surgical procedures, which also raises the risk of oversedation, especially older patients. Furthermore, some patients may take their own prescription medications or illicit drugs in addition to what is prescribed while hospitalized. Thus, AG-ACNPs need to closely monitor for oversedation and be ready to reverse these agents and support the patient with noninvasive ventilation, and potentially intubation and mechanical ventilation.

Fast Facts

AG-ACNPs must be able to rescue hospitalized patients who develop respiratory depression from conscious sedation. The reversal agent for opioids is naltrexone (Narcan), and the reversal agent for benzodiazepines is flumazenil (Romazicon).

Cholinergic Overdose

Cholinergic overdose symptomatology can be remembered with the mnemonic DUMBBELLSS or SLUDGE to help recall the cholinergic toxidrome (see Table 16.7).

Table 16.6

Clinical Presentations of Toxidromes With Examples of Agents

Toxidrome	Vital signs	Mental status	Eye exam	Additional findings	Examples of agents
Anticholinergic	Hyperthermia, tachycardia, hypertensive, tachypnea	Hypervigilant, agitated (mad as a hatter), hallucinating	Mydriasis (blind as a bat)	Dry, flushed skin (dry as a bone, red as a beet), urinary retention	Atropine, antihistamines, TCAs, scopolamine, antispasmodics, jimson weed, psychedelic mushrooms
Cholinergic	Bradycardia, tachycardia, hypertension	Confused, coma	Miosis	Salivation, lacrimation, urination, diaphoresis/diarrhea, GI upset, emesis (SLUDGE)	Organophosphates, carbamate pesticides, cholinesterase inhibitors, nerve agents, physostigmine
Opioid	Hypothermia, bradycardia, hypotension, bradypnea	CNS depression, coma	Miosis	Hyporeflexia, pulmonary edema	Opioids (morphine, oxycodone, hydrocodone, hydromorphone, fentanyl, codeine, methadone, heroin, etc.)
Sedative/hypnotic	Hypothermia, bradycardia, hypotension, bradypnea	CNS depression, confusion, coma	Miosis	Hyporeflexia	Benzodiazepines, nonbenzodiazepine GABA agonists, barbiturates, chloral hydrate, alcohols
Sympathomimetic	Hyperthermia, tachycardia, tachypnea	Agitated, hyperalert, paranoia	Mydriasis	Diaphoresis, tremors, hyperreflexia, seizures	Cocaine, amphetamines, pseudoephedrine, phenylephrine, ephedrine
Serotonergic	Hyperthermia, tachycardia, hypertension, tachypnea	Confused, agitated, coma	Mydriasis, ocular clonus	Tremor, myoclonus, diaphoresis, hyperreflexia, trismus, rigidity, muscular hypertonicity	MAOIs, SSRIs, buspirone, tramadol, dextromethorphan
Neuroleptic malignant syndrome	Hyperthermia, tachycardia, hypertension, tachypnea, arrhythmias	Agitated, delirious	Oculogyric crisis (rare)	Trismus, dystonia, ataxia, parkinsonism, neuroleptic malignant syndrome	Haloperidol, olanzapine, quetiapine, chlorpromazine, promethazine, prochlorperazine, fluphenazine, perphenazine

CNS, central nervous system; Miosis, constricted pupils; Mydriasis, dilated pupils.

Table 16.7

Mnemonics for Cholinergic Overdose

DUMBBELLSS	SLUDGE
D—Diarrhea	S—Salivation
U—Urination	L—Lacrimation
M—Miosis	U—Urination
B—Bronchorrhea	D—Diaphoresis and/or diarrhea
B—Bronchospasm	E—Emesis
E—Emesis	
L—Lacrimation	
L—Lethargy	
S—Salivation	
S—Seizures	

Fast Facts

Ingestion of cholinergic agents can be lethal. An easy way to recall the most serious symptoms that lead to death is to remember the "Killer Bs": bronchorrhea and bronchospasm.

Serotonin Syndrome

Serotonin syndrome (SS) is another challenging toxidrome to diagnose (see Tables 16.8 to 16.10). This toxidrome is important to highlight, as many commonly prescribed medications can cause SS alone or in combination with other agents. Additionally, these agents when combined with certain commonly prescribed antimicrobial agents can also trigger SS in hospitalized patients. Signs and symptoms of SS mimic the inflammatory response and are commonly mistaken for sepsis in hospitalized patients. Sepsis should always be excluded initially and then consider SS secondarily.

Fast Facts

Commonly prescribed medications can cause serotonin syndrome alone or in combination with other agents.

Table 16.8

Agents Associated With Serotonin Syndrome by Mechanism of Action

Agents	Mechanism of action
Monoamine oxidase inhibitors (MAOI): phenelzine, tranylcypromine, isocarboxazid, moclobemide, safinamide, selegiline, rasagiline Antibiotics: linezolid and tedizolid Others: methylene blue, procarbazine, Syrian rue	Decreased serotonin breakdown
Antidepressants – Selective serotonin reuptake inhibitors (SSRI): citalopram, escitalopram, fluoxetine, fluvoxamine, paroxetine, sertraline – Serotonin-norepinephrine reuptake inhibitors (SSNRI): duloxetine, milnacipran, venlafaxine – Tricyclic antidepressants: clomipramine, imipramine Herbals: St. John's wort Opioids: meperidine, buprenorphine, tramadol, tapentadol, dextromethorphan Antiepileptics: valproate, carbamezapine Antiemetics: ondansetron, granisetron, metoclopramide	Decreased serotonin reuptake
Tryptophan, lithium, fentanyl Illicit substance: lysergic acid diethylamide (LSD)	Increased serotonin precursors or agonists
Central nervous system stimulants: amphetamines Anorectics: fenfluramine, dexfenfluramine, phentermine Illicit substance: methylenedioxymethamphetamine (MDMA), cocaine	Increased serotonin release
Antibiotics: erythromycin, ciprofloxacin Antifungal: fluconazole Antiretroviral: ritonavir	CYP2D6 and CYP3A4 inhibitors

Toxins and Antidotes

AG-ACNPs can see routinely prescribed medications be accidentally or purposely overingested or overdosed upon. The AG-ACNP must be able to easily identify the reversal agent and dosing to rescue the patient from untoward effects, including organ failure and possible death (see Table 16.11).

In summary, AG-ACNPs will encounter substance-use disorders on a daily basis. Additionally, ingestions, whether intentional or accidental, are common. Patients may take their own medications in addition to those administered in the hospital. Patients also may receive anesthetics, sedatives, and other narcotics while hospitalized, as such the AG-ACNP

Table 16.9

Signs and Symptoms of Serotonin Syndrome

Mild	Moderate	Life-Threatening
Autonomic dysfunction: – Mild tachycardia – Mydriasis – Diaphoresis Altered mental status: – Anxiety – Restlessness – Insomnia Neuromuscular excitation: – Tremor – Hyperreflexia – Myoclonus	Autonomic dysfunction: – Tachycardia – Hyperthermia (<40 °C, <104 °F) – Hypertension – Hyperactive bowel sounds, diarrhea, nausea, vomiting Altered mental status: – Agitation – Disorientation Neuromuscular excitation: – Opsoclonus – Spontaneous or inducible clonus	Autonomic dysfunction: – Tachycardia – Hyperthermia (>40 °C, >104 °F) – Hypertension Altered mental status: – Confusion – Delirium – Coma Neuromuscular excitation: – Rigidity – Respiratory failure – Tonic-clonic seizure

Table 16.10

Serotonin Syndrome Treatment

Mild	Moderate	Severe
– Observe 6+ hours – remove causative agents – IVF for hydration/ diuresis – Benzos for agitation	– Admit to hospital with telemetry – Mild treatment plus: – Cyproheptadine PO/NGT 12 mg load, then 2 mg Q2 h if symptoms continue – Olanzapine 10 mg SL – Chlorpromazine 50–100 mg IM	– Admit to ICU – Moderate treatments plus: – Sedatives – IV antihypertensive agents – Cooling measures – Muscle relaxants (dantrolene) – Intubation/paralysis (vecuronium)

Table 16.11

Specific Toxin and Adult Dosing of Antidotes

Drug/agent	Antidotes	Doses
Acetaminophen	N-acetylcysteine	140 mg/kg PO or IV over 1 hour, then 70 mg/kg over 1 hours Q4 hour × 5 doses, then reassess toxin clearance, PT/INR and transaminases
Anticholinergics	Physostigmine	2 mg over 4 minutes, may repeat Q1–Q2 hours PRN

(continued)

Table 16.11

Specific Toxin and Adult Dosing of Antidotes (*continued*)

Drug/agent	Antidotes	Doses
Benzodiazepine	Flumazenil	.5 mg over 30 seconds; may repeat Q30–Q60 minutes
Beta-blockers	Glucagon	5 mcg/kg IV over 1–2 minutes up to 10 mg max; follow with infusion of half to full initial dose
Calcium-Channel Blockers	10% Calcium Chloride Dextrose and insulin	1–2 gm over 5 min (CVC preferred); may repeat 25 gm IV as D50% (50 mL) & .5–1 unit/kg bolus followed by .5–1 unit/kg per hour infusion
Cholinergic	Atropine Pralidoxime	.02 mg/kg IV or IM 1–2 g IV infusion (10–20 mg/mL) over 15–30 min, repeat in 1 hour if necessary and Q12 hours PRN
Coumadin	Phytonadione, Fresh frozen plasma Prothrombin complex concentrate (PCC)	10 mg IV daily × 3 days 15 mL/kg (roughly 3 units FFP for therapeutic INR) INR 2 - <4 = 25 units/kg maximum 2,500 units; INR 4–6 = 35 units/kg maximum 3,500 units; INR >6 = 50 units/kg maximum 5,000 units
Cyanide	Hydroxocobalamin**S odium nitrite Sodium thiosulfate, or	70 mg/kg over 15 minutes 300 mg over 2–5 minutes 12.5 gm bolus
Digoxin	Digibind	10–20 vials over 30 minutes for acute empiric dosing or base on serum digoxin levels
Ethylene glycol, methanol	Fomepizole** Ethanol	15 mg/kg/dose IV load over 30 minutes, then 10 mg/kg Q12 hours × 4 doses, then 15 mg/kg Q12 hours PRN till nontoxic. 10 mL/kg of 10% vol/vol solution, then continuous infusion of 1.5 mL/kg till nontoxic; double rate during dialysis.
Heparin	Protamine sulfate	1–1.5 mg per 100 USP units of heparin; not to exceed 50 mg; monitor APTT 5–10 minutes after dose then in 2–8 hours

(*continued*)

Chapter 16 Patients With Substance-Use Disorders and Toxicological Issues

Table 16.11

Specific Toxin and Adult Dosing of Antidotes (*continued*)

Drug/agent	Antidotes	Doses
Insulin	Glucose	D50% 50 mL bolus IV; consider D10% infusion and titrate to glucose levels
Iron	Deferoxamine	5 mg/kg per hour continuous infusion and titrate to 15 mg/kg/hr as tolerates total daily dose 6–8 gm
Isoniazid, hydrazine	Pyridoxine	5 gm IV
Lead	Dimercaprol	75 mg/m² Q4 hours, first dose to precede edetate calcium disodium (CaNa2 EDTA)
	CaNa2 EDTA	1,500 mg/m² by continuous infusion
	Succimer (DMSA)	10 mg/kg PO Q8 hours for 5 days, then 12 hours for 14 days
Methemoglobinemia	Methylene blue 1%	1–2 mg/kg IV over 5 minutes with 30 mL flush; may repeat 1 mg/kg ×1
Methotrexate	Folinic acid (leucovorin)	100 mg/m² over 15–30 minutes Q3–Q6 hours with resolution of bone marrow toxicity
Neuroleptics	Bromocriptine	5 mg Q12 hours increase to effect, as high as 10 mg Q6 hours
	Dantrolene	3–10 mg/kg over 15 minutes with oral doses of 25–600 mg/d to maintain response
Opioids	Naloxone	.5 mg IV with repeat dosing Q15 minutes to reversal of respiratory depression (can be given IM or ETT)
Organophosphates	Atropine	1–2 mg IV, double Q3–Q5 min until bronchorrhea resolves
	Pralidoxime (2-PAM)	1–2 gm over 30 minutes, then up to 500 mg/hr; Alternatively, 30 mg/kg IV (IM, SC if no IV access) over 20 minutes; follow by 4–8 mg/kg/hr maintenance IV infusion; IM: 600 mg IM ×3 doses; administer each dose 15 minutes apart for mild symptoms, or in rapid succession for severe symptoms
Sulfonylureas	Octreotide	50 mcg SC Q6–Q12 hours

(*continued*)

Table 16.11

Specific Toxin and Adult Dosing of Antidotes (*continued*)

Drug/agent	Antidotes	Doses
TCAs	Sodium bicarbonate	50 mEq per dose to address acidemia and/or ECK signs of sodium channel blockade (150 mEq and KCl 40 mEq in 1-L D5W. Serum pH 7.5–7.55.)
Valproic acid	L-carnitine	Clinically ill: 100 mg/kg IV over 30 minutes (max 6 gm), then 15 mg/kg Q4 hours Clinically well: 100 mg/kg PO per day (max 3 gm) divided Q6 hours

**Preferred.

must know how to reverse the effects of narcotics and benzodiazepines to rescue patients who may develop respiratory depression.

References

Hargraves, D., White, C., Frederick, R., Cinibulk, M., Peters, M., Young, A., & Elder, N. (2017). Implementing SBIRT (Screening, Brief Intervention and Referral to Treatment) in primary care: Lessons learned from a multipractice evaluation portfolio. *Public Health Reviews*, 38(1), 1–11.

Kuo, K. *Toxic ingestions*. www.learnpicu.com/toxidromes

Murray, E., Walthall, L., & Wise, K. R. (2017). Drug overdose and withdrawal. In S. J. McKean, J. J. Ross, D. D. Dressler, D. B. Scheurer (Eds.), *Principles and Practice of Hospital Medicine* (2nd ed., pp. 2057–2069). McGraw Hill Education.

Rasimas, J. & Sinclair, C. M. (2017). Assessment and management of toxidromes in the critical care unit. *Critical Care Clinics*, 33(3), 521–541.

Turner, A. H., Nguyen, C., Kim, J., & McCarron, R. (2019). Differentiating serotonin syndrome and neuroleptic malignant syndrome. *Current Psychiatry*, 18, 30–36.

Pralidoxime. Medscape. https://reference.medscape.com/drug/protopam-2pam -antidote-pralidoxime-343744

Rubinsky, A. D., Dawson, D. A., Williams, E. C., Kivlahan, D. R., & Bradley, K. A. (2013). AUDIT-C scores as a scaled marker of mean daily drinking, alcohol-use disorder severity, and probability of alcohol dependence in a U.S. general population sample of drinkers. *Alcoholism: Clinical and Experimental Research*, 37(8), 1380–1390.

Saunders, J. B., Aasland, O. G., Babor, T. F., De La Fuente, J. R., & Grant, M. (1993). Development of the alcohol-use disorders identification test (AUDIT): WHO collaborative project on early detection of persons with harmful alcohol consumption-II. *Addiction*, 88(6), 791–804.

Skinner, H. A. (1982). The drug abuse screening test. *Addictive Behaviors, 7*(4), 363–371.

Smith, P. C., Schmidt, S. M., Allensworth-Davies, D., & Saitz, R. (2009). Primary care validation of a single-question alcohol screening test. *Journal of General Internal Medicine, 24*(7), 783–788.

Vitesnikova, J., Dinh, M., Leonard, E., Boufous, S., & Conigrave, K. (2014). Use of AUDIT-C as a tool to identify hazardous alcohol consumption in admitted trauma patients. *Injury, 45*(9), 1440–1444.

Villalobos-Gallegos, L., Pérez-López, A., Mendoza-Hassey, R., Graue-Moreno, J., & Marín-Navarrete, R. (2015). Psychometric and diagnostic properties of the Drug Abuse Screening Test (DAST): Comparing the DAST-20 vs. the DAST-10. *Salud Mental, 38*(2), 89–94.

17

Older Adult Patients

Older adult patients comprise the majority of hospitalized patients. Additionally, the frail elder population continues to grow, as people are living well into their 90s and beyond. AG-ACNPs must constantly be aware of normal physiologic changes, and pharmacokinetics and pharmacodynamics associated with prescribing for this population. A foundational tenet of prescribing in the older adult population is to "start low and go slow." Avoid inappropriate medications in hospitalized older patients, as they are at greater risk for delirium, which can increase complications, length of stay, and mortality.

In this chapter, you will learn

- normal physiologic changes associated with aging,
- pharmacokinetics in the aging population,
- tips for prescribing for older hospitalized patients,
- drugs to avoid with older patients, and
- causes of falls in the older population.

Medication Reconciliation

AG-ACNPs need to be well versed with the physiologic changes occuring within the aging process. Differentiating between normal physiologic changes and pathological processes can be difficult. Many times, pathological changes are contributed to normal aging, thus delaying diagnosis and treatment of disease processes (see Table 17.1).

The medication reconciliation process can be challenging, as older adults have multiple medical problems, multiple prescribers, new diagnoses, recent hospitalizations, and any transition of care can change

Table 17.1

Physiologic Changes With Aging

Organ system	Changes	Implications
Neurological	↓ Autoregulatory capabilities Brain atrophy Short-term memory loss	↑ Susceptibility to injury May not recall taking pain medications
Pulmonary	↓ Vital capacity ↓ Forced expiratory volume Smaller alveolar surface area ↓ Chest wall compliance	↓ Respiratory reserve
Cardiac	↓ Cardiac output ↓ Sensitivity to catecholamines	↓ Cardiac reserve VS may not reflect severity of illness
Renal	↓ GFR ↓ Renal mass	Baseline renal impairment ↑ Risk of CIN ↑ Susceptibility to fluid overload Reduced clearance of certain medications
Hepatic	↓ Hepatic function	↓ Clearance of certain medications
GI	↓ Pain sensation ↑ Laxity of ABD wall Difficulty swallowing/chewing	Potential for significant intra-abdominal process without peritoneal signs May not be able to ingest certain medications
Immune	Impaired immune response	↑ Risk of infection
Musculoskeletal	Loss of muscle mass Osteoporosis	↑ Risk of fractures

medication regimens. Each medication reconciliation process requires the NP's full attention. Routinely practice the "brown bag" method to review each medication, dosage, administration, timing, and adherence to prescription. The "brown bag" method involves the patient or family bringing in all prescribed and over-the-counter medications and supplements they currently take and compare these bottles to their medication lists. Invite caregivers to participate. Do not rely solely on the medication list in the electronic health record or on pharmacy data; rather, integrate these lists and compare with the patients and their "brown bag" of medications.

Tips for Prescribing for Older Adults

- Minimize or eliminate medications when possible.
- Perform thorough medication review to ensure accuracy.
- Stop medications that are not indicated or have no clear benefit.
- When prescribing, be cognizant of physiological changes and pharmacokinetic effects that occur with aging. See Table 17.2.

Table 17.2

Pharmacokinetics in Aging

Process	Physiological change	Pharmacokinetic effect
Distribution	Decreased total body mass, increased proportion of body fat	Increased volume of distribution of highly lipid-soluble drugs
	Decreased proportion of body water	Decreased volume of distribution of hydrophilic drugs
	Decreased plasma albumin, disease-related increase in α1 acid glycoprotein	Changed % of free drug, volume of distribution, and measured levels of bound drugs
	Altered relative tissue perfusion	
Metabolism	Reduced liver mass, liver blood flow, and hepatic metabolic capacity	Accumulation of metabolized drugs
Excretion	Reduced glomerular filtration, renal tubular function, and renal blood flow	Accumulation of metabolized drugs

- All prescriptions must have a clear indication.
- Avoid drugs that have known deleterious effects in older patients. (See Beers criteria.)
- Start low, go slow. Start with 1/4 to 1/2 dose; can always add more but can't get it back once it's been given.
- Use nonpharmacological treatments such as heat, cold, compression, splints, and so forth.
- Limit the number of people prescribing for each patient if possible.
- Avoid treating adverse drug reactions with additional drugs.
- Check creatinine clearance, not just creatinine, and dose accordingly.
- Use caution with benzos due to decreased hepatic function; avoid if at all possible due to the risk of delirium.
- Maximum Acetaminophen (Tylenol) dose 3 gm/d
- Delirium—determine if delirium is medication related versus a new acute problem.
- Align management plan to the older patient's comorbidities; physical, cognitive, and physiological function; and personal preferences.

Fast Facts

When prescribing for the older population, start low and go slow! You can always add more, but you can't get it back once it's been given!

BEERS Criteria

The BEERS criteria are medications or types of medications that are "potentially inappropriate" for ages >65. There are three categories of medications on the BEERS list:

- Potentially inappropriate medication in older adults.
- Potentially inappropriate medication in older adults due to drug-disease or drug-syndrome interactions that may exacerbate a disease.
- Potentially inappropriate medication in older adults: drugs to be used with caution in older adults.

Consider avoiding these agents, as they have a higher risk of side effects (see Table 17.3). They may not work as well and should be replaced with safer or more effective medications or nonpharmacological interventions.

Table 17.3

BEERS Criteria: Medications to Avoid in Older Adults

Neurological

Analgesics
- Meperidine
- NSAIDs
  - Aspirin >325 mg/d
  - Diclofenac
  - Diflunisal
  - Etodolac
  - Fenoprofen
  - Ibuprofen
  - Indomethacin
  - Ketoprofen
  - Ketorolac
  - Meclofenamate
  - Mefenamic acid
  - Meloxicam
  - Nabumetone
  - Naproxen
  - Oxaprozin
  - Piroxicam
  - Sulindac
  - Tolmetin

Anticholinergics
- Brompheniramine
- Carbinoxamine
- Chlorpheniramine
- Clemastine
- Cyproheptadine
- Dexbrompheniramine
- Dexchlorpheniramine
- Dimenhydrinate
- Diphenhydramine (oral)

Benzodiazepines
Alprazolam
Estazolam
Lorazepam
Oxazepam
Temazepam
Triazolam
Chlordiazepoxide
Clonazepam
Clorazepate
Diazepam
Flurazepam
Quazepam

Nonbenzodiazepine, benzodiazepine receptor agonists hypnotics (e.g., Z-drugs)
- Eszopiclone
- Zaleplon
- Zolpidem

Antispasmodics
- Atropine (excludes ophthalmic)
- Belladonna alkaloids
- Clidinium-chlordiazepoxide
- Dicyclomine homatropine (excludes ophthalmic)
- Hyoscamine
- Methscopolamine
- Propantheline
- Scopolamine

(continued)

Table 17.3

BEERS Criteria: Medications to Avoid in Older Adults (*continued*)

Neurological

- Doxylamine
- Hydroxyzine
- Meclizine
- Promethazine
- Pyrilamine
- Triprolidine

Antiparkinsonian agents

- Benztropine (oral)
- Trihexyphenidyl

Antidepressants

- Amitriptyline
- Amoxapine
- Clomipramine
- Desipramine
- Doxepin >(6 mg/d)
- Nortriptyline
- Paroxetine
- Protriptyline

Barbiturates

- Amobarbital
- Butabarbital
- Butalbital
- Mephobarbital
- Pentobarbital
- Phenobarbital
- Secobarbital

Antithrombotics

- Dipyridamole—oral short-acting

Antipsychotics

- First-generation (conventional)
- Second-generation (atypical)

Muscle relaxants

- Carisoprodol
- Chlorzoxazone
- Cyclobenzaprine
- Metaxalone
- Methocarbamol
- Orphenadrine

Cardiovascular

Peripheral alpha-1 blockers:

- Doxazosin
- Prazosin
- Terazosin

Central alpha-agonists

- Clonidine

Other CNS alpha-agonists

- Guanabenz
- Guanfacine
- Methyldopa
- Reserpine (>.1 mg/d)

Other cardiac agents

- Disopyramide
- Dronedarone
- Digoxin (for 1st-line treatment of atrial fibrillation)
- Nifedipine (immediate release)
- Amiodarone

(*continued*)

Table 17.3

BEERS Criteria: Medications to Avoid in Older Adults (*continued*)

Endocrine

- Methyltestosterone
- Testosterone
- Desiccated thyroid
- Estrogens with or without progestins
- Growth hormone
- Megestrol

Sulfonylureas (long-acting)

- Chlorpropamide
- Glimepiride
- Glyburide

Gastrointestinal

- Metoclopramide
- Mineral oil (orally)
- Proton pump inhibitors

Renal/genitourinary

- Desmopressin

Infectious Disease

- Nitrofurantoin

Fast Facts

Always refer to the Beers criteria prior to prescribing for older patients.

FALLS AND SYNCOPE

Falls in the older population require specific exploration to determine if it was a mechanical fall, meaning they recall tripping over an object, or if they had a syncopal episode. Older adults can experience syncope for a variety of reasons, including orthostatic hypotension from dehydration and hypovolemia; infection, which can lead to sepsis; cardiac arrhythmias, including brady- or tachyarrhythmias; aortic insufficiency; stroke or hypoperfusion due to atherosclerotic arteries; hypotension due to medications; seizures; or, less frequently, autonomic dysfunction. The causative factor should be identified during the hospitalization so as to prevent further syncope or risk for additional harm, including death or rehospitalization.

In summary, older adults, especially frail ones, require considerable attention to prescribing practices. Pay special attention to pharmacokinetics and pharmacodynamics due to the pathophysiological changes that occur during the aging process. Start low and go slow! Refer to the Beers criteria prior to prescribing, and avoid these agents when at all possible. Reduce the number of medications or dosages when risks outweigh benefits. Evaluate the role of medications when patients report falls or syncope.

References

Alpert, J. S. (2019). Syncope in the Elderly. *The American Journal of Medicine*, *132*(10), 1115–1116.

American Geriatrics Society Beers Criteria® Update Expert Panel. Fick, D. M., Semla, T. P., Steinman, M., Beizer, J., Brandt, N., Dombrowski, R., DuBeau, C. E., Pezzullo, L., & Epplin, J. J. (2019). American Geriatrics Society 2019 updated AGS Beers Criteria® for potentially inappropriate medication use in older adults. *Journal of the American Geriatrics Society*, *67*(4), 674–694.

McKearney, K., & Coleman, J. J. (2020). Prescribing medicines for elderly patients. *Medicine*, *48*(7), 463–467.

Milton, J. C., Hill-Smith, I., & Jackson, S. H. (2008). Prescribing for older people. *BMJ*, *336*(7644), 606–609.

18

Care of Veterans

Veterans of the armed forces are a special population and warrant special attention. Many who served do not consider themselves veterans, especially those who served during peace times, did not see combat, or were in the National Guard. Regardless, they have distinct needs due to physical or psychological injuries from the experiences and exposures that the average person doesn't encounter. Many of these individuals seek care outside the Veterans Health Administration (VHA) healthcare system, thus AG-ACNPs need to be able to meet their specific needs.

In this chapter, you will learn

- questions pertinent to patients who have served in the armed services,
- specific illnesses/syndromes that are specific to each war, and
- management of veterans with PTSD.

VETERANS

The Veterans Health Administration (VHA) reports that <20% of all veterans in America receive care from the VHA healthcare system, and 40% of service-connected disabled veterans do not use the VHA for their care. Statistically, providers are already taking care of veterans in every practice setting. Thus, asking patients about service in the armed services is critical to getting to know your patient and providing holistic, patient-centered care. Military service, whether in peacetime or during war, is an occupation fraught with stressors, toxic exposures, hazards, and safety risks not commonly encountered in the civilian population. Healthcare providers in the private sector must be aware of their patients' military histories and the related health concerns resulting from that military service. This starts with a thorough history of their service in the armed forces, including:

- Have you or someone close to you ever served in the military?
  - When did you serve in the armed forces?
  - Which branch?
  - What did you do while you were in the military?
  - Were you assigned to a hostile or combative area?
  - Did you experience enemy fire, see combat, or witness casualties?
  - Were you wounded, injured, or hospitalized?
  - Did you participate in any experimental projects or tests?
  - Were you exposed to noise, blasts, chemicals, gases, demolition or munitions, pesticides, or other hazardous substances?
- Have you ever used the VHA for healthcare?
  - When was your last visit to the VHA?
  - Do you have a service-connected disability or condition?
  - Do you have a VHA primary care provider?

Fast Facts

Every patient should be asked if they've ever served in the armed forces. This includes the Coast Guard and Army or Air National Guard. Simply asking if they are a veteran misses the opportunity to include these other populations who have the same exposures.

Illness Syndromes by War

Certain health concerns are consistent through every war, while others are unique to each specific conflict. The most common conditions for all conflicts include:

- musculoskeletal injuries with chronic pain
- posttraumatic stress disorder (PTSD)
- dental needs
- hearing loss

Conditions Unique to Specific Conflicts:

- World War II: cold injury (Europe); peptic ulcer disease (PUD) and gastrointestinal complaints
- Korea: cold injuries (e.g., frostbite)
- Vietnam: Agent Orange–exposure illnesses

- amyloidosis
- chronic B-cell leukemia
- chloracne (or similar acneform disease)
- diabetes mellitus type 2
- Hodgkin disease
- ischemic heart disease
- Multiple Myeloma
- non-Hodgkin lymphoma
- Parkinson disease
- early-onset peripheral neuropathy
- porphyria cutanea tarda
- prostate cancer
- cancers of the lung, larynx, trachea, and bronchus
- soft-tissue sarcomas (other than osteosarcoma, chondrosarcoma, Kaposi sarcoma, or mesothelioma)

- Persian Gulf War I: unexplained medical symptoms (Gulf War Syndrome)
  - Symptoms may include, but are not limited to, abnormal weight loss, fatigue, cardiovascular disease, muscle and joint pain, headache, menstrual disorders, neurological and psychological problems, skin conditions, respiratory disorders, and sleep disturbances.
  - chronic fatigue syndrome
  - fibromyalgia
  - functional gastrointestinal disorders:
    - a group of conditions marked by chronic or recurrent symptoms related to any part of the gastrointestinal tract
    - examples include irritable bowel syndrome, functional dyspepsia, and functional abdominal pain syndrome

- Operation Enduring Freedom (Afghanistan), Operation Iraqi Freedom (Iraq), Operation New Dawn (Iraq, post-"end of combat operations in August 2010"):
  - traumatic brain injury/polytrauma
  - musculoskeletal injuries
  - mental-health disorders
  - ill-defined conditions
  - nervous system (hearing loss)
  - GI (dental needs)
  - endocrine/nutrition
  - injury/poisoning
  - respiratory

- Southwest Asia (including Iraq) or Afghanistan: may experience infectious diseases while on active duty or develop symptoms later, including:
  - malaria

- brucellosis
- *Campylobacter jejuni*
- *Coxiella burnetii* (Q fever)
- *Mycobacterium tuberculosis*
- Nontyphoidal *Salmonella*
- shigella
- visceral Leishmaniasis
- West Nile Virus

Diagnosis and Management of PTSD

Most cases of PTSD are seen in combat veterans, along with many victims of sexual assault. Nearly 23% of female veterans reported being sexually assaulted while serving in the military. Symptoms usually begin within 3 months but can be delayed for months or more longer (see Tables 18.1 and 18.2). The classic symptoms of PTSD following exposure

Table 18.1

PTSD Stressors

PTSD stressors	PTSD triggers
Physical: • injury • noise • temperature • sleep deprivation • diet • austere conditions • toxic agents • infectious agents • multiple immunizations • blast wave/head injury Psychological: • anticipation of combat • combat trauma • noncombat trauma • separation from family/home • deprivation Psychosocial: • marital/parenting issues • social functioning • occupational/financial concerns • risk of redeployment • spiritual/existential	• Lack or loss of power/control • Transitions and routine/schedule disruption • Feelings of vulnerability and rejection • Feeling threatened or attacked • Sensory overload • Sights, sounds, smells, physical surroundings, and situations (fireworks) • Emotional state of mind (terror, rage, grief, adrenaline rush) • Exposure to traumatic events that include an element of victimization, racism, or catastrophic losses • Anniversary dates such as holidays and times of the year that have meaning from time in war zone • Media exposure to war zone–like events • Music that elicits feelings related to those experienced during war time • Significant losses, such as death of a loved one, divorce, separation, financial or job losses, serious illnesses, loss of bodily functions or parts, or imminent death • Conflicts with authority figures, including medical, governmental, religious, or supervisors

PTSD, posttraumatic stress disorder.

Table 18.2

Interventions to Treat PTSD

Outpatient	Inpatient
• Cognitive therapy, cognitive behavioral therapy* • Exposure therapy* • Stress inoculation training* • Present-centered therapy • Interpersonal psychotherapy • Psychoeducation* • Narration (oral, written, fictional)* • Eye movement desensitization and reprocessing • Complementary and alternative modalities (meditation, acupuncture, Reiki, yoga) • Pet/dog therapy • Benzodiazepines are contraindicated	• If currently on medication for PTSD, restart as soon as possible • Consider psychiatry consultation • Always coordinate with PCP's office so provider is aware • Recommend use of sertraline and paroxetine (FDA-approved); fluoxetine and venlafaxine also recommended but off label • Prazosin (Minipress) for treatment of nightmares • Avoid divalproex, tiagabine, guanfacine, risperidone, benzodiazepines, D-cycloserine • Benzodiazepines are strongly discouraged unless they cannot be avoided due to severe hypoxic respiratory failure or alcohol-withdrawal interventions. • Consider dexmedetomidine (Precedex) for sedation needs

*A-level recommendation.
FDA, Food and Drug Administration; PCPs, primary care physicians; PTSD, posttraumatic stress disorder.

to an extreme traumatic stressor that involves a threat to the physical integrity of themselves or others include:

- hyperarousal/hypervigilance
- intrusive memories and reexperiencing (flashbacks)
- avoidance responses: withdrawal or distancing
- trouble sleeping
- trouble concentrating
- memory problems
- relationship problems
- aggression
- self-destructive behavior (self-harm or substance abuse)
- low sense of self-worth and hopelessness

Substance Use in Veterans

Veterans with PTSD commonly self-treat their symptoms with opioids, sedatives, alcohol, or substances including marijuana and other illicit substances. Thus, concomitant substance-use disorder is common among veterans. Veterans should be screened for substance-use disorder. Refer to chapter on substance use/toxicology for additional details on screening, brief intervention, and referral to treatment (SBIRT) intervention.

Fast Facts

Nearly 20% of service members reported binge drinking on a weekly basis, which was higher among veterans with exposure to combat.

In summary, veterans of the armed forces have unique needs and don't always seek care through the VHA system. Thus, AG-ACNPs need to first identify which patients are veterans and discuss their specific service-related healthcare needs. Customize the care of these patients in the context of these needs. Seek expert guidance from VHA providers to aid in meeting their needs.

References

U.S. Department of Veterans Affairs. (2018). *Gulf War Veterans' Medically Unexplained Illnesses.* www.publichealth.va.gov/exposures/gulfwar/medically-unexplained-illness.asp

U.S. Department of Veterans Affairs. (2019). *PTSD: National Center for PTSD.* www.ptsd.va.gov/professional/index.asp

The Management of Posttraumatic Stress Disorder Work Group. (2017). *VA/DOD clinical practice guideline for the management of posttraumatic stress disorder and acute stress disorder.* www.healthquality.va.gov/guidelines/MH/ptsd/VADoDPTSDCPGFinal012418.pdf

Platoni, K. Warning Signs, Triggers, and Coping Strategies for Iraqi War Veterans Patriot Outreach. https://patriotoutreach.org/warning-signs.html#1

Juergens, J. (2021, 24 March 2021). *Veterans and Addiction. Addictions Center.* www.addictioncenter.com/addiction/veterans

19

Obstetrical Patients

Educational programs and scope of practice for AG-ACNPs do not historically include obstetrical care. However, increasingly, obstetrical patients are requiring critical care services for a variety of conditions. To ensure AG-ACNPs remain within their scope of practice, a collaborative approach with the obstetrical team is required for optimal patient outcomes. Ongoing consultation with obstetrical physicians, midwives, nursing, pharmacy, and respiratory therapy should occur routinely throughout every shift.

In this chapter, you will learn

- normal physiologic changes with pregnancy,
- drugs to use and avoid with pregnant patients, and
- to recognize and treat common obstetrical emergencies.

ICU admission criteria for pregnant patients is neitherclearly defined nor universally accepted. Pregnant women may be admitted to ICU for pregnancy-related conditions, medical or surgical reasons not related to pregnancy, and underlying diseases that worsen during pregnancy. While obstetrical nurses routinely manage the problems listed in Table 19.1, these patients are specifically admitted to the ICU for advanced monitoring, management of arterial lines, telemetry, neurological concerns, respiratory or cardiac failure, and general closer observation. Critical care nurses possess experience, intuition, and act swiftly to respond to patient deterioration, which in turn improves patient outcomes. Therefore, AG-ACNPs who work in ICU must know the physiologic changes related to pregnancy to best respond to these conditions when in the ICU (see Table 19.2).

Table 19.1

Indications for Admission of Obstetrical Patients to ICU

Pregnancy-related conditions	Nonpregnancy-related	Disorders worse in pregnancy
• Hemorrhage • Infections/sepsis • Preeclampsia/eclampsia • Amniotic fluid embolism • HELLP syndrome • Aspiration	• Trauma • Asthma • Diabetes • Autoimmune diseases (e.g., SLE, myasthenia gravis)	• Anemia • Congenital heart disease • Rheumatic heart disease • Pulmonary hypertension • Renal failure • Autoimmune disorders

HELLP, hemolysis, elevated liver enzymes, and low platelets; SLE, systemic lupus erythematosus.

Table 19.2

Physiological Changes in Pregnancy

System	Changes	Impact
Cardiovascular	↓ Peripheral vascular resistance ↑ Heart rate ↓ Arterial pressure Increased cardiac output	Masks initial signs of sepsis ↑ Hypoperfusion Uteroplacental circulation cannot autoregulate, thus dependent on maternal circulation
Blood	↑ Plasma volume ↑ Red cell volume Anemia	Greater reduction of oxygen supply to tissues
Respiratory	↑ Tidal volume ↑ Respiratory rate ↑ Minute ventilation by 30–40% ↓ Residual volume	Decreased ability to respond to metabolic acidosis Impaired oxygenation
Renal	↑ Renal blood flow, GFR ↓ Creatinine levels Ureteral dilation and ↓ Ureteral pressure due to smooth muscle relaxation Flaccid bladder ↑ Intravesical pressure due to pregnant uterus weight ↑ Vesicoureteral reflux ↑ Renal plasma flow ↑ Glomerular filtration rate ↓ Urea and creatinine Asymptomatic bacteriuria	Even normal levels can signify renal compromise Delays identification of renal injury secondary to sepsis Favorable to pyelonephritis

(continued)

Table 19.2

Physiological Changes in Pregnancy (*continued*)

System	Changes	Impact
Gastrointestinal	↓ Tone of lower esophageal sphincter ↓ Muscle tone across the GI tract ↓ Perfusion of gastric mucosa Delayed gastric emptying Diaphragm elevation by the uterus Changes in bile composition ↑ Production of pro-inflammatory cytokines by Kupffer cells	↑ Risk of aspiration ↑ Risk of bacterial translocation ↑ Risk of aspiration pneumonia ↑ Risk of cholestasis, hyperbilirubinemia, and jaundice
Hematological	↑ Leukocyte count ↓ Platelet count ↑ Factors VII, VIII, IX, X, XII, von Willebrand and fibrinogen ↓ Protein S ↓ Fibrinolytic activity	Leukocytosis is unreliable indicator of sepsis ↑ Risk of thrombotic events Increased risk of DIC
Genital	Uteroplacental circulation cannot autoregulate ↓ Vaginal pH ↑ Glycogen in vaginal epithelium	Maternal infection can easily affect the fetus ↑ Risk of chorioamnionitis

DIC, disseminated intravascular coagulation; GFR, glomerular filtration rate.

General Principles

The average perinatal mortality rates continue at an unacceptably high rate, ranging from 5.37 to 7.60 per 1,000 for all age groups, except for maternal age over 40, which has a mortality rate of 9.86 per 1,000, and the highest mortality rate is observed in the non-Hispanic Black population at 10.66/1,000. These rates have remained unchanged since 2014. Given this significant concern for maternal and fetal health, a multidisciplinary approach to critically ill pregnant patients is essential to ensure the best outcomes for both the mother and infant. Collaboration among intensivists, obstetricians, AG-ACNPs, midwives, pediatrician or neonatologist, nurses from both critical care and obstetric areas, as well as pharmacists and other supporting team members is vital. Treatment should focus on stabilization of both the mother and fetus. In circumstances when the fetus is over 24 weeks of gestation, the ICU team should be prepared for an emergent delivery and/or Cesarean. If/when emergent delivery is needed, the AG-ACNP manages the mother, while the obstetrical team manages the delivery.

Medications

AG-ACNPs need to carefully weigh the risks and benefits of any drug used with pregnant women. The Food and Drug Administration (FDA) narrative classification provides a summary of evidence or lack of evidence. The FDA classifies medications into three categories: (1) pregnancy, (2) lactation, and (3) females and males of reproductive potential. Within each category is a description of risk summary, clinical considerations, and additional data. This categorization provides the prescriber with more narrative information upon which to assess risk to the patient.

Fast Facts

Avoid use of any medication in pregnancy that is not absolutely necessary!

Drug Resources

The InfantRisk Center Health Care Mobile Resource from iMedical Apps contains critical safety information on most prescription and over-the-counter medications, vitamins, and supplements. It provides evidence-based, quick reference for pregnancy and breastfeeding safety (www.imedicalapps.com/2020/06/infantrisk-center-health-care-mobile-resource). Additionally, the InfantRisk Center has a website for providers and patients, including a worldwide hotline for providers to call with questions about medication safety.

The drugs and lactation database by LactMed contains information on medications and other chemicals that breastfeeding mothers may encounter. Peer-reviewed, evidence-based information on levels in breast milk, possible adverse effects to the infant, and suggestions for alternative therapies are included in this online resource (www.ncbi.nlm.nih.gov/books/NBK501922) (see Tables 19.3 to 19.5).

Fast Facts

Routinely consult the obstetrical team and pharmacist about any medications prior to use.

Venous Thromboprophylaxis

Obstetrical patients are at a higher risk for venous thromboembolism (VTE). Thromboprophylaxis guidelines by the American Congress of Obstetricians and Gynecologists (ACOG) recommend mechanical thromboprophylaxis for all patients undergoing Cesarean delivery. Pharmacological prophylaxis with low-molecular-weight heparin (LMWH) or unfractionated heparin (UFH) for high-risk thrombophilia, any prior VTE event, or a family history of VTE thrombophilia.

Table 19.3

Drugs in Pregnancy

Generally considered safe in pregnancy	Drugs to avoid during pregnancy
Acetaminophen	ACE inhibitors
Amoxicillin with clavulanic acid	Aminoglycosides
Beta-blockers	Angiotensin receptor blockers
Bisacodyl	Aspirin
Calcium carbonate	Amiodarone
Cephalosporins	Barbiturates
Chlorpheniramine	Bismuth subsalicylate
Colace	Calcium channel blockers
Clindamycin	Chloramphenicol
Dextromethorphan	Clarithromycin
Digoxin	Diethylstilbestrol
Diphenhydramine	Diazepam
Dobutamine	Enalapril
Famotidine	Fluoroquinolones
Furosemide	Ketamine
Guaifenesin	Ketoconazole
Hydralazine	Loratadine
Loperamide	Metronidazole
Heparin—low molecular weight (LMWH)	Misoprostol
• Enoxaparin	Nitroprusside
• Dalteparin	NSAIDs
• Tinzaparin	Omeprazole
Heparin (unfractionated)	Pseudoephedrine
Ivermectin	Sodium bicarbonate
Labetalol	Spironolactone
Magnesium hydroxide	Statins
Metamucil	Streptomycin
Meclizine	Sulfonamides
Milrinone	Tetracyclines (doxycycline, minocycline)
Nicardipine	Thiazide diuretics
Nifedipine	Tigecycline
Penicillin	Theophylline
Phosphodiesterase inhibitors	
Prostacyclin	
Simethicone	
Senna	

ACE, angiotensin-converting enzyme; NSAIDs, nonsteroidal anti-inflammatory drugs.

Avoid use of warfarin due to teratogenic effects. Patients with a history of, or who are at risk of, VTE may also be changed to UFH prior to delivery as needed to balance the risks of bleeding and thrombosis at the time of delivery and to minimize any impact on the fetus.

Table 19.4

ICU Analgesics and Sedatives for Obstetrical Patients

Drug (category)	Adverse effects	Safety
Opioids • Fentanyl • Morphine • Hydromorphone	• Respiratory depression • Risk of newborn withdrawal syndrome	• Notify pediatrician/ neonatologist of opioid use
Propofol	• Hypotension • (Higher doses [2.8 mg/kg] can result in lower Apgar scores, muscle hypotony, and depressed neuromuscular activity)	• Limited data
Dexmedetomidine	• Increased myometrial contraction in rats	Limited data
Benzodiazepines • Midazolam • Lorazepam	• Respiratory depression • Floppy infant syndrome • Withdrawal syndrome in the newborn	• Considered contraindicated in pregnancy • Potential use in eclamptic seizures

Table 19.5

Antimicrobial Agents in Pregnancy

Considered safe in pregnancy	Avoid during pregnancy
Antibiotics/Antiviral: • Aztreonam • Azithromycin • Penicillin • Cephalosporins • Clindamycin • Gentamicin • Macrolides • Nitrofurantoin • Vancomycin Antivirals: • Acyclovir • Oseltamivir Antifungals: • Obstetrical patients experience increased vaginal candidiasis due to increased hormones. Topical azoles are first line in the first trimester	• Clarithromycin • Quinolones • Tetracyclines (doxycycline, minocycline) • Tigecycline • Amphotericin • Oral fluconazole: associated with an increased risk of spontaneous abortions and stillbirths due to teratogenicity in high dosage

Sepsis/Septic Shock in Obstetrical Patients

Sepsis can be challenging to recognize in the pregnant patient due to the physiological changes associated with pregnancy. Septic shock is most commonly due to pyelonephritis, chorioamnionitis, and endometritis. Management of septic shock is congruent with any nonpregnant patient and should follow the sepsis clinical practice guidelines. Antibiotics commonly used in pregnant septic patients include ampicillin, clindamycin, and metronidazole. Therapy should continue for 7 to 10 days. De-escalation is difficult due to the polymicrobial nature of these infections. Outcomes of sepsis in pregnant patients is typically better due to the nature of a generally healthy and younger population without comorbid conditions.

Critical Care Obstetrical Emergencies

Obstetrical emergencies routinely require admission to critical care units for ongoing management. Table 19.6 lists a few of the more common conditions that the AG-ACNP may be engaged to comanage along with intensivists and obstetric and pediatric teams.

Fast Facts

For severe preeclampsia, eclampsia, HELLP syndrome, and any fetal distress, urgent delivery is indicated.

POSTPARTUM COMPLICATIONS

Postpartum complications can occur and can be serious enough to warrant an ICU admission. For any postpartum patient in ICU, the AG-ACNP should note the date of last delivery, since physiologic changes of pregnancy and common postpartum complications have been overlooked, causing delays in treatment. Delays in recognition and treatment along with associated maternal morbidity and mortality has led to recommendations to increase training for ED and ICU staff related to postbirth events.

Postpartum patients are at high risk for venous thromboembolisms (VTE) for up to a month postdelivery. Maintain a high index of suspicion for patients who present with shortness of breath, leg swelling, and tachycardia. Additionally, patients can develop sepsis and/or septic shock due to endometritis from retained placenta during birth. Lastly, mastitis can also complicate recoveries of women admitted to the ICU during the postpartum period.

In summary, obstetrical patients are complex to manage due to changes in physiology, pregnancy-specific pathology, and maternal

Table 19.6

Obstetrical Emergencies, Diagnostic Criteria, and Treatments

Obstetric emergency	Diagnostic criteria	Treatment

Severe preeclampsia	Eclampsia:
	• BP >140/90 on two readings over 4 hours apart or >160/110 on two readings minutes apart; proteinuria >300 mg/24 hours
	Severe preeclampsia is preeclampsia with any of the following:
	• Platelet count <100,000 uL
	• Creatinine >1.1 mg/dL or twice the patient's baseline
	• AST or ALT >twice upper limit of normal or RUQ pain
	• Pulmonary edema
	• CNS symptoms—headache, changes in vision
		• BP control with IV pushes of labetalol or hydralazine or infusion of labetalol or nicardipine Intravenous magnesium
		  • Load of 4–6 gm IV over 15–30 minutes followed by 2 gm/hour
		  • Recurrent seizures 2 gm over 10–15 minutes
		• Watch for signs of magnesium toxicity: patellar reflexes, somnolence, respiratory difficulty, cardiac dysrhythmias
		• To reverse magnesium: calcium gluconate 10 mL over 10 minutes

Eclampsia	Severe preeclampsia (as above) plus seizures or coma	• BP control as above • Intravenous magnesium • Monitor for signs of magnesium toxicity, and treat as above • Deliver the fetus
Hemorrhagic shock (can be due to uterine atony; placenta previa, accreta, increta, or percreta; uterine rupture; surgical and urogenital tract trauma)	• Note: Overt signs of bleeding may be absent or misinterpreted as normal physiological changes with pregnancy. Shock signs: • Sinus tachycardia • Tachypnea • Anxiousness, restlessness • Pallor, cool skin, diaphoresis • Oliguria or anuria • Hypotension	• Volume resuscitate with blood, plasma, platelets, and cryoprecipitate • Warm the patient • ABG to assess acid–base status • Place a urinary catheter • Bimanual massage • Uterotonics: oxytocin infusion • Manual exploration to remove retained products of conception • Weight risk/benefit of tranexamic acid or recombinant factor VIIa • Interventions: balloon tamponade, uterine artery embolization, operative interventions

(continued)

Table 19.6

Obstetrical Emergencies, Diagnostic Criteria, and Treatments (*continued*)

Obstetric emergency	Diagnostic criteria	Treatment

HELLP syndrome (hemolysis, elevated liver enzymes, and low platelets)	Subjective but not specific: nausea, vomiting, headache, general malaise requires laboratory evaluation:
	• Hemolysis:
	  • Schistocytes on blood smear
	  • Elevated indirect bilirubin
	  • LDH >600 IU or bilirubin >1.2 mg/dL
	  • Low serum haptoglobin (≤25 mg/dL)
	• AST >70 U/L
	• Platelets <100,000/mm³
		• Deliver the fetus

Amniotic fluid embolism	Abrupt onset with rapid deterioration • Dyspnea • Profound hypoxemia • Profound hypotension • Cardiac dysrhythmias • Cyanosis • Pulmonary edema or ARDS • Altered mental status and/or seizures • Disseminated intravascular coagulation and hemorrhage	• Immediate delivery of the fetus • Treatment depends on the severity of illness and capabilities of the institution • Intubate and mechanically ventilate • Vasopressor and inotropic support • Consider inhaled nitric oxide or prostacyclins • Intraaortic balloon pump, ventricular assist devices, ECMO, or cardiopulmonary bypass
Peripartum cardiomyopathy	• Idiopathic cardiomyopathy • Develops near the end of pregnancy/within months of delivery • Absence of an identifiable cause • LV systolic dysfunction (dilated or nondilated) • EF <45%	• Urgent cardiology consultation for workup, comanagement, device therapy, transplantation evaluation • IV furosemide for preload reduction • Vasodilators for afterload reduction • With shock: inotropic support with dobutamine or milrinone

(*continued*)

Table 19.6

Obstetrical Emergencies, Diagnostic Criteria, and Treatments (*continued*)

Obstetric emergency	Diagnostic criteria	Treatment
		• For compensated state beta blockade • For low EF or evidence of VTE—anticoagulate. • ACEi are contraindicated during pregnancy; recommended in postpartum period

ABG, arterial blood gases; ALT, alanine aminotransferase; ARDS, acute respiratory distress syndrome; AST, aspartate aminotransferase; CNS, central nervous system; ECMO, extracorporeal membrane oxygenation; EF, ejection fraction; LDH, lactate dehydrogenase; LV, left ventricular; RUQ, right upper quadrant; VTE, venous thromboembolism.

and fetal considerations. Care of these patients requires intense interprofessional collaboration with nursing, obstetrics and pediatric teams, and intensivists, pharmacists, and consultants. Routine referencing of evidence-based resources should be done prior to any prescribing for pregnant or lactating patients.

References

Buscher, M. & Edwards, J. H. (2020). Obstetric Emergency Critical Care. In *Emergency Department Critical Care*, Springer, pp. 503–532.

Kaur, M., Singh, P. M., & Trikha, A. (2017). Management of critically ill obstetric patients: A review. *Journal of Obstetric Anaesthesia and Critical Care*, 7(1), 3.

Chen, J., Cox, S., Kuklina, E. V., Ferre, C., Barfield, W., & Li, R. (2021). Assessment of incidence and factors associated with severe maternal morbidity after delivery discharge among women in the U.S. *JAMA Network Open*, 4(2), e2036148. https://doi.org/10.1001/jamanetworkopen.2020.36148

Gregory, E. C. W., Drake, P., & Martin, J. A. (2018). *Lack of change in perinatal mortality in the United States, 2014–2016*. NCHS Data Brief, No 316. National Center for Health Statistics.

(2006). *Drugs and Lactation Database (LactMed) [Internet]*, National Library of Medicine (U.S.). www.ncbi.nlm.nih.gov/books/NBK501922

IV

Special Considerations for Advanced Practice Acute Care Nursing

20

Ethical and Legal Issues

AG-ACNPs commonly encounter conflicts while caring for acutely and critically ill patients and their families. The majority of such conflicts are easily resolved with effective communication and enhanced education. Unresolved conflicts can lead to ethical dilemmas and even legal challenges.

In this chapter, you will learn

- the definitions of common ethical terms,
- indications for ethics committee consultations,
- to differentiate between capacity and competency,
- the elements of informed consent, and
- to distinguish between claims made and occurrence malpractice insurance policies.

ETHICAL TERMS

Autonomy: The right to self-govern.

Beneficence: The moral obligation to promote goodness or benefit to the patient. Provide care that maintains or improves health status, decreases disability, and eases physical pain and suffering.

Nonmaleficence: To refrain from doing harm.

Justice: To strive for fair distribution of resources.

Veracity: To convey the truth. Being honest and telling the truth is related to the principle of autonomy.

Fidelity: To be faithful; accurate in details and exactness. Fidelity is to keep one's promises. Nurse practitioners must be faithful and true to professional codes of conduct and standards of care and responsibilities.

Accountability: An obligation to accept responsibility or to account for one's actions.

INDICATIONS FOR ETHICS CONSULT

The Joint Commission requires hospitals to have a process to handle ethical situations. Ethics committees are commonly interprofessional in nature, including physician, nursing, social work, legal counsel, clergy, ethicist, and/or others determined by the hospital. Consultation with the hospital ethics team can occur for ANY reason. Typical reasons for consultation include the following issues or concerns:

- advance directive or surrogate decision-making
- "Do Not Resuscitate" orders
- brain-death criteria/pronouncement
- capacity/informed consent
- isolated and/or incapacitated patient
- futility or demand for ineffective treatments
- discharge or placement issues
- maternal/fetal concerns
- medical errors
- pain-management issues
- refusal of recommended treatments/interventions
- research ethics
- resource allocation
- transplantation matters
- withdrawal of life-sustaining therapies, including ventilators and nutritional support
- cultural/ethnic/religious
- breach of confidentiality
- communication issues
- quality-of-life concerns
- dispute/conflict

  - within the family
  - between staff
  - staff-family
  - staff-patient
  - denial of condition by patient or family
  - attitude of provider about treatment(s)

The legal surrogate decision-maker varies from state to state. In some states, a guardian has the highest authority to make medical decisions, whereas in other states a healthcare proxy or durable power of attorney for healthcare is the legally accepted medical decision-maker (MDM). The AG-ACNP is responsible for identifying the legal decision-maker who can make surrogate decisions on behalf of the patient, if the patient does not have the capacity or competency to make their own decisions.

If no surrogate is identified, states commonly define who and in what order relatives or next of kin can be the MDM. Commonly, the order is first the spouse, followed by adult children, parents, and siblings. When the order is not clear or when challenges arise, consult the hospital's legal team for clarification and assistance. For adolescents who are considered mature minors, please consult with specific state laws, adolescent health specialists, and institutional legal teams, as this population presents with significantly more complex situations.

Types of proxy decision-making include substituted judgment and best interest standard. Substituted judgment occurs when the surrogate applies the knowledge of patient preferences to make medical decisions for the patient. When the patient's preferences are not known, the best interest standard would apply. This situation occurs when the surrogate acts in the best interest of the patient. When MDMs do not follow substitute judgment, or do not act in the best interest of the patient, which can occur when there are secondary gains, consult the hospital's legal team or ethics team for guidance.

INFORMED CONSENT

Informed consent is the process in which patients agree to accept medical interventions after adequate disclosure of the nature of the interventions. Treatment options are explained in layman's terms to the patient and/or their designee. The risks and benefits of and alternatives to the proposed interventions are explained to the patient so the patient can decide upon an intervention or treatment plan. To make informed decisions, the patient must have capacity to participate in this process. If a patient does not have capacity, the surrogate decision-maker must be engaged in the process. Elements of informed consent:

- Informed consent is a patients' right.
- Informed consent requires that the patient have the capacity to participate
- Without capacity, patients need a surrogate decision-maker.
- Care can be provided under emergency presumption.

Competency

Medical competency is a legal term that is the key to rational decision-making. Our laws assume every adult is mentally competent until a court decides otherwise. Thus, only a judge can deem a person incompetent to make their own decisions. This typically requires a series of neurological and psychological exams performed by a neuropsychologist to guide this judgment.

Capacity

In hospitalized patients, capacity can change from day to day, and even hour to hour sometimes, depending on the status of medical conditions, medications or anesthetics, delirium, and so forth. NPs should perform an assessment to determine capacity when decisions need to be made (see Exhibit 20.1).

Exhibit 20.1

Questions to Ask During an Evaluation of Medical Decision-Making Capacity

Questions to determine the patient's ability to understand treatment and care options:

- What is your understanding of your condition?
- What are the options for your situation?
- What is your understanding of the benefits of treatment, and what are the odds that the treatment will work for you?
- What are the risks of treatment, and what are the odds that you may have a side effect or bad outcome?
- What is your understanding of what will happen if nothing is done?

Questions to determine the patient's ability to appreciate how that information applies to their own situation:

- Tell me what you really believe about your medical condition.
- Why do you think your doctor has recommended (specific treatment/test) for you?
- Do you think (specific treatment/test) is best for you? Why or why not?
- What do you think will actually happen to you if you accept this treatment? If you don't accept it?

Questions to determine the patient's ability to reason with that information in a manner supported by the facts and the patient's own values:

- What factors/issues are most important to you in deciding about your treatment?
- What are you thinking about as you consider your decision?
- How are you balancing the pluses and minuses of the treatments?

(continued)

Exhibit 20.1

Questions to Ask During an Evaluation of Medical Decision-Making Capacity (*continued*)

- Do you have confidence that you are receiving appropriate treatment from your provider?
- What do you think will happen to you now?

Questions to determine the patient's ability to communicate and express a choice clearly:

- You have been given a lot of information about your condition. Have you decided what medical option is best for you right now?
- We have discussed several choices. What do you want to do?

The elements of informed consent include competence, disclosure, understanding, and consent. Patients must have the capacity to make the medical decision. AG-ACNPs must disclose the risks, benefits, and alternatives regarding the specific diagnostic test, treatment, or procedure. The patient must be able to comprehend the information provided and grant voluntary consent without coercion or duress.

During medical emergencies, when a patient cannot consent due to the critical nature of the situation, consent is implied. In other words, it is assumed the patient would consent if they could, when the alternative is death or severe morbidity. This concept protects the provider from being charged with battery. To deem a procedure or intervention emergent, the AG-ACNP should document the rationale for this decision in the procedure note. If a second provider is present and concurs that it is an emergent intervention, the AG-ACNP should also document this agreement of the second provider.

Fast Facts

While we may not always agree with a patient's or family's decision, we must respect the decision. It is helpful to seek to understand the reasoning behind the decisions.

MEDICAL ERRORS

Disclosure of medical errors is expected when harm is caused to a patient. This should be done as soon as facts are known and upon consultation with the risk-management department. Open disclosure, by stating facts that are currently known, and the status of ongoing investigations should occur as quickly as possible. Do not share suppositions of how something may have happened or point fingers as to who or what may have occurred. Simply convey the facts in an empathetic, nondefensive manner. Disclosure and apology for the error can reduce malpractice litigation; conversely, failure to disclose can increase litigation. State laws are evolving to support apology for medical errors. Patients and families want to know how the institution is responding so as to prevent others from incurring similar harms.

MALPRACTICE INSURANCE

NPs are increasingly being named as defendants in lawsuits; thus, all NPs need to ensure they have malpractice insurance coverage. Most hospitals provide malpractice insurance as part of the compensation package. Medical malpractice insurance covers several expenses associated with defending and settling suits, including paying damages if the NP is found liable. Covered costs include attorney fees, court costs, arbitration costs, settlement cost s, and punitive and compensatory damages as well as medical damages. Malpractice insurance does not cover liability from acts committed while under the influence of drugs or alcohol, sexual misconduct, criminal acts, and inappropriate changes to medical records.

The decision to purchase your own, separate malpractice policy is a very personal decision. NPs should understand the pros and cons of having a separate policy and ask questions of the employer's policies to make an informed decision as to whether to procure an individual policy (see Table 20.1).

When choosing insurance options, recognize that claims can be filed years after the treatment occurred. Understanding this when deciding

Table 20.1

Pros/Cons of an NP Having Their Own Malpractice Insurance Policy

Pros	Cons
• The NP will have his/her own legal counsel with expenses covered.	• The NP may be drawn into the lawsuit or kept in a lawsuit longer in hopes of drawing from the NP's insurance. Whether or not an NP has a policy will be identified during the discovery phase.
• The NP may be covered for incidents that occurred out of the employment setting (e.g., if volunteering).	
• The NP may be able to purchase higher limits than the hospital.	• It's a significant expense.
• For occurrence policies, the NP will have coverage if he/she leaves the employer.	

upon types of policies is important. "Claims made" policies provide coverage if the policy is in effect when the treatment occurred and when the suit is filed, whereas "occurrence policies" cover claims for care that took place during the period of coverage regardless if the claim is filed after the policy lapses. Some policies offer "tail coverage," which extends coverage after the policy ends, commonly for about 5 years. Consider adding this coverage when changing to a new position or getting ready to retire.

Questions to ask of an employer's or hospital's policy before deciding upon procuring your own policy:

- Is it a commercial policy, or is the organization self-insured?
- For commercial policies, are there any exclusions or circumstances that aren't covered? What is the company's financial stability rating?
- If self-insured, are there limits to what the hospital will pay for damages, attorney fees, expert witness fees, and so forth? What are these limits?
- Are any NP activities excluded from coverage, or are there requirements for supervision of NP practice that the policy requires?
- Is it an occurrence policy or claims made policy? If the latter, inquire as to who pays for the tail coverage and how much it will cost if not covered by the hospital.

NPs are advised to purchase individual coverage if:

- The employer policy is claims made and the hospital won't pay or the NP can't afford the tail coverage.
- You perform NP services outside of your employment.
- When the hospital policy covers you only under certain conditions and you can't meet all the conditions.
- The insurance company has a rating <A−.
- The employer policy limits are below $1 million per incident.

In summary, AG-ACNPs will continue to encounter legal and ethical dilemmas throughout the tenure of their careers. Recognition of the issues and mobilization of resources are key to resolving the situation. To that end, recognizing moral distress and activating resources to support yourself are equally important.

References

Armstrong, K. & Silverman, R. D. (2017). Medical-legal concepts: advance directives and surrogate decision-making. In S. J. McKean, J. J. Ross, D. D. Dressler, & D. B. Scheurer (Eds.), *Principles and Practice of Hospital Medicine* (2nd ed., pp. 224–230). McGraw Hill Education.

Barstow, C., Shahan, B., & Roberts, M. (2018). Evaluating medical decision-making capacity in practice. *American Family Physician*, 98(1), 40–46. www.aafp.org/afp/2018/0701/p40.html#afp20180701p040-b12

Buppert, C. (2018). *Nurse practitioner's business practice and legal guide* (6th ed.). Jones & Bartlett.

Fins, J. J., McCarthy, M. W., & Limehouse, W. (2017). Common indications for ethics consultation. In S. J. McKean, J. J. Ross, D. D. Dressler, & D. B. Scheurer (Eds.), *Principals and Practice of Hospital Medicine* (2nd ed., pp. 217–223). McGraw Hill Education.

O'Connor, M. F. & Dalton, A. K. (2017). Ethics, palliative, and end-of-life care. In G. Frendl & R. D. Urman (Eds.), *Pocket ICU* (2nd ed.). Wolters Kluwer.

Schaffer, A. C. (2017). Medical malpractice. In S. J. McKean, J. J. Ross, D. D. Dressler, & D. B. Scheurer (Eds.), *Principles and Practice of Hospital Medicine* (pp. 231–239). McGraw Hill Education.

21

Palliative Care

Palliative care is specialized medical care for people with life-limiting illness. The goals of palliative care are to improve symptom management, assess and support caregiver/family needs, and assist with care coordination. Palliative care consultations are appropriate for many hospitalized patients to provide extra support for the patient and family. NPs should be discussing palliative care with patients and families when death within a year would not be surprising, and consider hospice when patients decline such that prognosis is likely to be death within 6 months. In fact, palliative care is increasingly being included in clinical practice guidelines as best practice.

In this chapter, you will learn

- overview of palliative care,
- key communication strategies,
- SPIKES protocol for family meetings,
- signs of the dying process, and
- symptom-management interventions.

OVERVIEW OF PALLIATIVE CARE

Palliative care is specialized medical care for people living with serious illness. The focus is on symptom management and relieving the stress of the illness in an effort to improve quality of life for the patient and the family. Palliative care differs from hospice in that it can assist with patient care regardless of prognosis and can be provided along with curative treatment. Communication surrounding a patient's goals of care is often a pivotal focus of palliative care.

Patients admitted to the hospital should have a goals-of-care discussion at the time of admission and any time there is a change in condition. This helps set realistic expectations for recovery with the patient and family. Start with an exploration of the health status over the last year. Elicit if there were multiple admissions. Has the patient returned to their previous level of health each time, or has there been a stepwise regression in overall health? Start goals-of-care discussions broadly to elicit the patient's perspective, and then narrow the discussion to specifics such as the need for intubation, CPR, or other life-sustaining interventions. Asking permission and offering your professional opinion on what you see as the best course of treatment are part of the shared decision-making process. All interventions should be decided based upon a risk/benefit analysis. Providers are not obligated to offer treatments that will not meet the goals of care or that are deemed futile.

Understand that a staged approach to these discussions over several days or meetings can be effective in shifting goals of care from curative to comfort measures. Communicating a consistent message will aid them in understanding the disease progression and/or failure to respond to treatments. Time-limited trials of treatments or interventions allow time for patients and families to come to terms and allow for evaluation of improvement or lack thereof.

COMMUNICATION SKILLS

Families are usually stressed when a loved one is hospitalized, especially if the course is tenuous and the patient is unstable or decompensating. Tips to communicating with families:

- Regularly communicate
  - Families want regular (daily) communication, from the same person if possible. Be sure to communicate changes in condition, and reassure them you will call if things change. If in doubt, make the call.
- Listen
  - Listen to see if the family understands the situation. Listening helps to establish trust and allows families to vent frustrations and fears. Ask about the patient's life, their values, and how the last few years of their life have been. Have they progressively deteriorated? Have they regained what was lost from the last admission?
- Provide psychological support
  - Recognize and acknowledge the emotion—put a name to it.
  - Validate the emotions with statements similar to this: "You seem distressed/angry/sad" or "This must be very difficult for you."

- Inform
  - Inform families about diagnoses, treatments, and whether goals of care are being met.
- Convey uncertainty
  - Do not be afraid to say "I don't know," but then get the answer for them (if at all possible).
- Care always continues
  - We never stop caring for the patient; we change the focus of the care from curative to comfort. We withdraw interventions, not care.
- Don't ask the family to decide
  - Rather, ask them "if (the patient) could know everything we just talked about, what would they choose for themselves?"

AG-ACNPs commonly communicate new diagnoses, describe treatments and interventions, provide updates to changes in conditions, explain prognosis, and discuss code status. Developing these skills takes time and repetition to refine. Thus, it's helpful to use a protocol to ensure a consistent pattern to the conversations. The SPIKES mnemonic is an available technique to organize a family meeting.

SPIKES PROTOCOL

- S = Set up
  - Prepare for the discussion.
  - Arrange for a private area.
  - Involve family/significant others with patient permission.
  - Sit down during the meeting; maintain eye contact.
  - Manage interruptions; that is, hand off the pager or phone to a colleague.

- P = Perception
  - Ask about the family's or patient's perception or understanding of their medical condition.

- I = Invitation
  - Ask how much the patient wants to know.
  - Ask who else the patient would like to be engaged in the conversation.

- K = Knowledge
  - Share your knowledge with the patient/family.
  - Prepare them to hear bad news: "I'm sorry, I need to share some bad news."
  - Avoid medical jargon.
  - Give information in small amounts, and check understanding before proceeding.

- E = Emotions
  - Address patient's/family's emotions with empathetic responses.

- S = Summarize/strategize
  - Assess understanding.
  - Ask if the patient is ready to discuss any decisions and treatment plan.
  - Create a treatment plan based on goals.

Fast Facts

Maintaining a consistent message about the patient's status among team members is key to developing trust. Be sure the messages from all members of the primary team, nursing team, and consulting teams are aligned. Patients and families who receive mixed messages from different team members can become frustrated and distrustful. Take time to discuss with each other before meeting with the patient and family to clarify the content of the message.

SIGNS OF THE DYING PROCESS

During family meetings, it can be helpful to elicit if the patient has experienced any of the following symptoms in the days/weeks/months. This can aid in helping the family understand the patient has been deteriorating over a period of time.

Weeks to months

- Anorexia
- Increased weakness
- Increased debility

Days to weeks

- Sleeping most of the day
- Decreasing urine output
- More staring, or withdrawal from environment
- Worsening dysphagia
- Near-death awareness (e.g., seeing or talking with deceased friends/ family)
- Transient improvement that is "rallying"; report that patient had a "really good day"
- Confusion, disorientation, delirium

Hours to days (actively dying)

- Irregular breathing
- Audible pulmonary or oral secretions (i.e., the "death rattle")
- Skin mottling, also known as livedo reticularis
- Ileus
- Minimal to no urine output
- Eyes open but not blinking

Minutes to hours

- Abnormal breathing—agonal respiratory pattern and/or jaw thrusting (guppy breathing)

END-OF-LIFE SYMPTOM MANAGEMENT

When a patient is converted to palliative care or even comfort measures, the AG-ACNP should evaluate all orders individually to determine whether each intervention contributes to the comfort of the patient. Consider withdrawal of the following therapies:

- ventilator support
- vasopressor support
- extracorporeal support (e.g., CRRT [continuous renal replacement therapy], intermittent hemodialysis, ECMO [extra corporeal membrane oxygenation], VAD [ventricular assist devices], IABP [intra-aortic balloon pump])
- defibrillator setting of AICD (Automatic internal cardiac defibrillator)
- antibiotics and curative pharmacotherapy
- supplemental oxygen, including BiPAP (bilevel positive airway pressure), CPAP (continuous positive airway pressure), and high-flow nasal cannula
- enteral and parenteral nutrition
- laboratory and radiology testing
- decrease frequency of vital signs or discontinue
- placement/removal of arterial lines, central venous catheters
- discontinue telemetry
- aggressive chest physical therapy
- thromboembolism prophylaxis

    Palliative and comfort measures commonly include:

- food/beverage the patient enjoys if able to take
- control of oral secretions
- analgesics
- sedatives
- anticonvulsants
- antipyretics
- nonsteroidal anti-inflammatory drugs
- prophylaxis for GI bleeding
- antiemetics

MEDICATION MANAGEMENT

Dyspnea/air hunger
    Opioids for dyspnea:

- Morphine 1 to 2 mg IV Q 2 hours or 3 to 5 mg PO Q 4 hours.

- Hydromorphone .2 mg IV Q 2 hours or 1 to 2 mg PO Q 4 hours.
- Oxycodone 2.5 to 5 mg PO Q 4 hours.
- Opioid tolerance: Increase baseline opioid dose by 25%.

Fast Facts

Not all patients who are placed on comfort measures require opioid infusions. Focus on symptom management. Explain to the family that these medications may hasten death, but the goal is symptom management. Purposefully hastening death is considered euthanasia.

Pain management

- Monitor for signs of pain, including vocalizations, diaphoresis, agitation, tachypnea, tachycardia.
- If unable to take oral agents, use:
    - IV opioids: morphine, fentanyl, hydromorphone, PRN dosing, PCAs, and infusions should be customized for each patient.
    - IV Ofirmev (Tylenol) 1,000 mg IV Q 8 hours.
    - IV ketorolac (Toradol) 30 mg IV × 1, then 15 mg IV Q 8 hours × 48 hours; use caution if actively bleeding.
    - Patches: fentanyl, lidocaine.

Fast Facts

Patients who have worsening pain, tremors, seizures, and hallucinations may have opioid neurotoxicity. Opioids may need to be reduced or rotated to a different medication.

Anxiolytics

- Lorazepam (Ativan) .5 to 1 mg PO or IV Q 1 hour till dyspnea controlled, then Q 4 to 6 hours.
- Midazolam (Versed) .2 to .5 mg IV Q 15 minutes till dyspnea controlled; can consider an infusion.
- Clonazepam (Klonopin) .25 to 5 mg PO Q 12 hours.

Agitation/delirium

- Haloperidol (Haldol) .5 to 2 mg PO, IV, or SC Q 6 hours can increase to hourly; maximum dose 20 mg in 24 hours.
- Olanzapine (Zyprexa) 2.5 to 5 mg PO or SL Q 12 hours and every 4 hours PRN; maximum 30 mg in 24 hours.
- Chlorpromazine (Thorazine) 25 to 50 mg PO, PR, or IV Q 8 hours and Q 4 hours PRN.

- Dexmedetomidine (Precedex) .2 to 1.2 mcg/kg/min infusion.

Management of oral secretions

- Oral suctioning and repositioning.
- Glycopyrrolate (Robinul) .1 to .2 mg IV Q 8 hours.
- Hyoscyamine (Anaspaz) .125 to .25 mg SL Q 6 to 8 hours.
- Scopolamine (Transderm Scop) 1.5 mg patch Q 72 hours.
- Atropine (Isopto Atropine) 1% ophthalmic drops administered SL Q 6 hours.

Antiemetic agents

- Ondansetron (Zofran) 4 to 8 mg PO or IV Q 8 hours.
- Prochlorperazine (Compazine) 5 to 10 mg PO or IV Q 6 hours.
- Promethazine (Phenergan) 12 to 25 mg PO or IV Q 6 hours.
- Metoclopramide (Reglan) 5 to 20 mg PO or IV Q 6 hours.
- Dexamethasone (Decadron) 4 to 20 mg PO or IV BID.
- Haloperidol (Haldol) .5 to 2 mg PO or IV Q 6 hours.
- Diphenhydramine (Benadryl) 25 to 50 mg PO or IV Q 6 hours.
- Lorazepam (Ativan) .5 to 2 mg PO or IV Q 6 hours.
- Scopolamine (Transderm Scop) 1.5 mg patch Q 72 hours.

Appetite stimulants for anorexia

- Dronabinol (Marinol) 2.5 to 7.5 mg PO TID.
- Prednisone (Deltasone) 5 mg PO TID.
- Dexamethasone (Decadron) 4 to 8 mg PO in divided doses.

In summary, any patient who a provider considers likely to die within the next 6 months to a year should be considered for a palliative care consult. By focusing on symptom management, patients can have improved quality of life for their remaining time. Clear communication surrounding goals of care can align patients with appropriate medical interventions.

References

Caissie, A. & Zimmermann, C. (2017). Communication skills for end-of-life care. In S. J. McKean, J. J. Ross, D. D. Dressler, & D. B. Scheurer (Eds.), *Principles and Practice of Hospital Medicine* (pp. 1733–1739). McGraw Hill Education.

Center to Advance Palliative Care. www.capc.org

Get Palliative Care. www.getpalliativecare.org/whatis

O'Connor, M. F. & Dalton, A. K. (2017). Ethics, palliative and end-of-life care. In G. Frendl & R. D. Urman (Eds.), *Pocket ICU* (2nd ed.). Wolters Kluwer.

Yeh, I. M. & Bernacki, R. E. (2017). Principles of palliative care. In S. J. McKean, J. J. Ross, D. D. Dressler, & D. B. Scheurer (Eds.), *Principles and Practice of Hospital Medicine* (2nd ed., pp. 1727–1732). McGraw Hill Education.

22

Moral Distress, Compassion Fatigue, Burnout, and Self-Care

Caring for multiple acutely and critically ill patients simultaneously can be mentally, physically, spiritually, and emotionally challenging. These challenges, combined with organizational constraints, limited resources, communication issues, complicated family dynamics, and end-of-life care, can wear on a provider's psyche, bringing a barrage of complex emotions ranging from satisfaction to grief to anger. How a provider responds to the daily challenges and emotions they face while caring for others affects the type of provider they become, resulting either in ruin or resilience. If one does not actively cultivate coping strategies to maintain resilience, moral distress, compassion fatigue, and burnout will develop and tint the provider's ability to be present with both the people they care for and their colleagues in the acute care setting. Developing and practicing self-awareness and compassionate self-care practices as a provider can ensure a long and healthy career.

In this chapter, you will learn

- to differentiate between moral distress, compassion fatigue, and burnout;
- self-care strategies to address moral distress, compassion fatigue, and burnout; and
- to differentiate between mindfulness and self-compassion.

MORAL DISTRESS

Moral distress is the multilayered response to tension a provider feels when they know the right thing to do but are unable to act on it due to organizational, procedural, or societal constraints (American Nursing Association, 2015). Moral distress arises when a provider feels that the ethically correct action differs from what he or she is tasked with doing. Examples include

- when policies or procedures prevent the NP from doing what they think is right;
- when a family desires an intervention(s) that the NP feels would do more harm than good; and
- when ongoing care is perceived as futile by the care team.

These situations present moral dilemmas and can make nurses feel powerless, anxious, and sad (see Tables 22.1 and 22.2). Nurses and NPs who work in critical care and emergency departments experience this more frequently.

COMPASSION FATIGUE

Compassion fatigue is the "cost of caring" for patients and their families and other loved ones who are in emotional pain. Compassion fatigue occurs when caregivers experience emotional and physical exhaustion due to bearing witness to others' suffering each day and feel powerless to help alleviate that suffering. This can lead to cynicism, emotional fatigue, or lack of focus in professionals who were previously devoted to their profession. When the caregiver is not able to replenish and rejuvenate themselves, they may begin to express that they are no longer able to care as much as they once did as a provider because they are just too worn down and tired.

Table 22.1

Signs and Symptoms of Moral Distress		
Emotional	Frustration Anger Anxiety Guilt	Sadness Powerlessness Withdrawal
Physical	Muscle aches Headaches Palpitations	Neck pain Diarrhea Vomiting
Psychological	Depression Emotional exhaustion Loss of self-worth	Nightmares Decreased job satisfaction Depersonalization of patients

Table 22.2

Causes and Resources of Moral Distress

	Causes	Resources
Self	• Witnessing patient suffering • Unnecessary treatments • Providing end-of-life care • False hope to patients/families • Care perceived as futile	• Share with a trusted colleague. • Connect with others for support. • Identify who can help. • Participate in professional development, such as palliative care or ethics education. • Seek help from clinical leaders and/or employee assistance program.
Unit	• Unhealthy work environment • Inadequate staffing • Ineffective communication • Incompetent or lazy colleague(s) • Bullying	• Pause after every patient death. • Conduct resilience rounds. • Create a mentoring program for new staff. • Identify ethics champions. • Recognize situations that cause distress. • Establish a committee to address distress. • Use AACN's Healthy Work Environment Assessment Tool.
Institution	• Limited resources • Financial constraints • Hospital policies • Lack of or ineffective communication	• Improve the work environment; use AACN's Healthy Work Environment standards. • Offer resources to support care teams. • Provide training on critical debriefing, resilience, and skilled communication. • Promote well-being of the team.

AACN, American Association of Critical-Care Nurses.

Fast Facts

Moral distress and compassion fatigue are generally seen as "warning signs" leading to burnout.

BURNOUT

When one experiences ongoing moral distress and compassion fatigue together and for an extended time, burnout is almost inevitable. Burnout is the physical, mental, and emotional exhaustion that occurs due to workplace stress and leads to poor engagement and depersonalization. Burnout does not always mean the caregiver lacks compassion for others. Internally, burnout impacts one's emotional, physical, and spiritual life, making one feel helpless, ineffective, and overwhelmed. Externally, burnout impacts job satisfaction, staff turnover, and culture, as well as employee and patient satisfaction scores. Burnout can be resolved with a change in position, or a change in the population the provider cares for. Burnout differs from compassion fatigue in that a change in job will not improve compassion fatigue. However, caregivers can concurrently experience compassion fatigue and burnout.

STEPS TO ADDRESSING MORAL DISTRESS

1. <u>Determine what you are experiencing</u>: Distinguish between moral distress, burnout, and compassion fatigue. Each can cause distress; however, each has different mitigation strategies.
2. <u>Gauge the severity of your distress</u>: Become familiar with the common symptoms, and rate your distress. This will help inform your mitigation strategies.
3. <u>Identify the causes of the distress</u>: Recognize the factors and situations that cause your distress; this will inform your next steps (see Table 22.3).
4. <u>Take action to move forward</u>: Consider all options to address your moral distress. Assess what is available to your unit or institution.

Recognizing signs and symptoms of moral distress in oneself and in fellow providers can help both to guide how to request support, and lead to change and growth on an individual or organizational level. Moral courage is developing inner strength to speak up despite the fear of consequences in order for change to occur. Moral resilience is the personal ability to restore and maintain one's integrity in response to moral distress, or simply put, the ability to bounce back in the midst of the many difficult scenarios one faces in the acute care setting.

Fast Facts

Moral courage is developing inner strength to speak up despite the fear of consequences. Moral resilience is the personal ability to restore and maintain one's integrity in response to moral distress.

Key characteristics of moral resilience:

- developing self-awareness
- cultivating mindfulness and creativity
- pursuing continued education in ethical challenges
- deepening moral compassion for others
- searching for meaning and growth in the midst of difficulty
- nurturing thoughtful action in one's self and others
- building and maintaining trust with colleagues

Table 22.3

Identifying, Preventing, and Coping with Moral Distress, Compassion Fatigue, and Burnout Tool

How do I identify compassion fatigue?	How do I prevent and cope with compassion fatigue?
Lack of empathy or compassion for others	
Reliance on unhealthy coping skills	
Impaired ability to care for others ("shutoff")	
Disruption of worldview (meaning/purpose)	
Diminished sense of enjoyment of work, cynicism	
How do I identify burnout?	*How do I prevent and cope with burnout?*
Withdrawal from family or friends	
Loss of interest in activities previously enjoyed	
Emotional and spiritual exhaustion (feeling irritable, hopeless, or helpless)	
Physical exhaustion (sickness, tiredness)	
Feelings of wanting to hurt yourself or others	
Change in appetite and/or weight	
Lack of self-care	
How do I identify moral distress?	*How do I prevent and cope with moral distress?*
Feelings of powerlessness	
Insomnia or nightmares	
Physical symptoms: GI issues, headaches, other	
Anxious or depressive symptoms	
Emotional lability extends from outburst to apathy	
Takes frustrations out on others with less authority	

SELF-CARE STRATEGIES

Self-care can be defined as "providing adequate attention to one's own physical and psychological wellness." Along with attention to physical and psychological wellness, emotional, social, and spiritual wellness also need to be considered when evaluating strategies that will work for you. Beginning with a self-assessment to take inventory of how you are doing in the following categories can be a good place to start:

Physical: Start with the basics, including a healthy diet, consistent meal times, regular exercise, quality sleep, and minimizing alcohol intake.

Psychological: There is a growing body of evidence supporting mindfulness as both a tool for stress relief and self-awareness. Additionally, use of mental-health services, including employee assistance programs, is beneficial to support you and the entire healthcare team.

Emotional: Set clear emotional boundaries between home and work; participate in regular bereavement practices to express grief that comes up in the acute care setting. Practice self-compassion and loving-kindness meditations, and practice gratitude each day.

Social: Spend time with family and friends, take vacations, engage in hobbies and leisure activities you enjoy, and so forth.

Spiritual: Spend time in nature; engage in religious practices such as prayer, meditation, or reflection.

You need to care for yourself so that you can care for others, be it patients and their loved ones or your colleagues. Give yourself permission to meet your own needs, especially when time is limited at work. Brief interventions, such as those in Tables 22.4 and 22.5, can provide a needed moment to recenter yourself in the midst of a busy day.

Brief self-care interventions can include giving yourself a soothing touch, speaking words of comfort to yourself, or taking a self-compassion break. The mindfulness and self-compassion exercises on the next few pages can be used to help ground yourself during a busy shift.

Self-compassion break: Acknowledge this is a moment of suffering, and accept that suffering is a part of life. Put your hand over your heart; feel the warmth and gentle touch of your hand on your chest. Repeat the following slowly and deliberately:

Table 22.4

Difference Between Mindfulness and Self-Compassion	
Mindfulness	**Self-compassion**
Experience acceptance	Accepting experiencer
What am I experiencing?	What do I need?
Feel your suffering with spacious awareness	Be kind to yourself when suffering

Table 22.5

Self-Comfort and Self-Compassion Exercises

A self-comfort moment:	Self-compassion affirmations:
• When you notice stress, close your eyes and take 2 to 3 long breaths. • Gently place your hand over your heart (alternatively wrap your arms around/hug yourself). • Feel the touch of your hands on your chest or arms. • Feel your chest rise and fall. • Linger with the feeling a moment.	Remind yourself of any/all of the following: • I accept myself as I am. • I am enough. • I am worthy of compassion. • I forgive myself and allow myself to feel inner peace. • I allow myself to make mistakes and to learn from those mistakes. • Let go of the old; make room for the new. • Today I treat myself with kindness. • Like any human I have strengths and weaknesses, and that's OK. • I am healing through self-compassion. • I give myself unconditional love.

- May I be kind to myself.
  - May I give myself the compassion that I need.
  - May I learn to accept myself as I am.
  - May I forgive myself.
  - May I be strong.
  - May I be patient.
- May I be kind to myself in this moment, at any moment, in every moment.
- May I accept this moment exactly as it is, any moment, every moment.
- May I accept myself exactly as I am in this moment, any moment, every moment.
- May I give myself all the compassion and courageous action that I need.

Mindfulness and loving-kindness meditation:

- Loving-kindness meditation: Promotes positive emotions, reduces negative criticism, increases compassion, activates empathy, enhances social connection and interpersonal attitudes.

  - May I be happy.
  - May I be free of physical pain and suffering.
  - May I be healthy and strong.
  - May I be able to live in this world happily, joyfully, and with ease.

The benefits of loving-kindness meditation include increased resilience, control over moods, willpower, sense of purpose, and empathy.

Gratitude practices

Practicing gratitude improves emotional well-being and improves the ability to cope with stress. Daily practice can impact physical health, relieve stress, improve sleep, and reducesdepression. Examples include gratitude journals, gratitude jars, written thank-you notes, sharing in person, and gratitude boards.

Fast Facts

Practice self-care daily. A healthy diet, exercise, minimizing alcohol consumption, self-compassion, and gratitude all work. When the job is simply too much or these strategies are insufficient, it's OK to ask for help from a professional. A session or two from the employee assistance program can do wonders for your mental health.

THE ROLE OF THE NP

As a leader on the care team, an NP needs to be observant, take the pulse of the team, and know what resources are available within their setting. When stress is noted, be present and listen to staff. Allow staff to openly share how they feel both mentally and physically without judgment. Acknowledge their experiences and feelings as valid, and respond in a kind and thoughtful manner. Encourage your team members to practice good self-care and normalize talking with a professional through your Employee Assistance Program when distress is chronically high. As you begin to become aware of your own moral distress, compassion fatigue, and burnout and begin to recognize the signs in others, you will be subtly building your own resilience.

In summary, nurses and nurse practitioners are at risk for moral distress compassion fatigue, and burnout. Perform regular check-ins with yourself and peers. Develop strategies to mitigate these adverse reactions to events we experience in our careers. Make self-care part of your daily routines, and enjoy a rich and rewarding career.

Resources:
Guided Meditations for Self-Compassion
https://self-compassion.org/category/exercises/#guided-meditations

Self-Compassion Exercises
https://self-compassion.org/category/exercises/#exercises

Self-Compassion Exercise for Caregivers
www.youtube.com/watch?v=jJ9wGfwE-YE&feature=youtube

Self-Compassion Break (mp3)
https://self-compassion.org/wp-content/uploads/2015/12/self-compassion.break_.mp3

Well-Being Initiative
www.nursingworld.org/thewellbeinginitiative

Healthy Nurse, Healthy Nation
www.hnhn.org

Nurse Suicide Prevention/Resilience
www.nursingworld.org/practice-policy/nurse-suicide-prevention

References

AACN. (2020, July 2020). *Addressing moral distress quick reference guide.* American Association of Critical Care Nurses. www.aacn.org/~/media/aacn-website/clincial-resources/moral-distress/recognizing-addressing-moral-distress-quick-reference-guide.pdf

ANA. (2001). *Code of ethics for nurses with interpretive statements.* Nursesbooks.org.

HNHN. (2017). *Moral distress: what it is and what to do about it.* Healthy Nurse, Healthy Nation. https://engage.healthynursehealthynation.org/blogs/8/531

Kornfield, J. (2008). *The art of forgiveness, loving kindness, and peace.* Bantam.

Mathieu, F. (2007). Running on empty: Compassion fatigue in health professionals. *Rehab & Community Care Medicine, 4,* 1–7.

Mathieu, F. (2019). *What is compassion fatigue?* www.tendacademy.ca/what-is-compassion-fatigue

McCue, C. (2010). Using the AACN framework to alleviate moral distress. *Online Journal of Issues Nursing, 16*(1), 9. https://doi.org/10.3912/OJIN.Vol16No01PPT02

Neff, K. & Germer, C. (2019). *The transformative effects of mindful self-compassion.* Mindful: Healthy Mind, Healthy Life. www.mindful.org/the-transformative-effects-of-mindful-self-compassion

Norcross, W. A., Moutier, C., Tiamson-Kassab, M., Jong, P., Davidson, J. E., Lee, K. C., Newton, I. G., Downs, N. S., & Zisook, S. (2018). Update on the UC San Diego healer education assessment and referral (HEAR) program. *Journal of Medical Regulation, 104*(2), 17–26.

Seppala, E. M., Hutcherson, C. A., Nguyen, D. T., Doty, J. R., & Gross, J. J. (2014). Loving-kindness meditation: A tool to improve healthcare provider compassion, resilience, and patient care. *Journal of Compassionate Health Care, 1*(1), 1–9.

Spadaro, K. (2020). *Effective tools for practicing self-compassion and self-care in the time of COVID-19.* American Nurses Association COVID-19 Webinar Series.

Winland-Brown, J., Lachman, V. D., & Swanson, E. O. C. (2015). The new "code of ethics for nurses with interpretive statements" (2015): Practical clinical application, Part I. *MedSurg Nursing, 24*(4), 268.

Index

Printed in the United States
by Baker & Taylor Publisher Services